Flatten Your Belly, Transform Your Life

The Proven Blueprint for Men to Lose Belly Fat Fast

Preface

Welcome to Flatten Your Belly, Transform Your Life: The Proven Blueprint for Men to Lose Belly Fat Fast. This book is more than a guide to shedding belly fat—it's a roadmap to reclaiming your health, energy, and confidence.

For many men, stubborn belly fat isn't just a cosmetic concern; it's a barrier to physical vitality and mental clarity. It's also linked to serious health risks like heart disease, diabetes, and low testosterone. In this book, I've distilled years of research, personal experience, and practical strategies into a step-by-step blueprint tailored specifically for men.

You'll learn the science behind effective fat loss, discover powerful workouts, and adopt nutritional habits that work for real, busy lives. Along the way, I'll help you break through the myths of quick fixes and teach you how to create sustainable results that last.

This is not about crash diets or endless hours in the gym—it's about smarter choices and a proven plan that fits into your life. My goal is to empower you to not only flatten your belly but also transform your mindset, health, and overall well-being.

Let this book be your guide as you take the first steps toward a healthier, stronger, and more vibrant you. The journey starts now!

— Arjun Thakur

About the Author

Arjun Thakur is a health and fitness enthusiast, lifestyle coach, and author passionate about transforming lives through science-backed strategies. With years of experience helping men reduce belly fat and achieve fitness goals, Arjun is a trusted guide in weight management and holistic health.

Combining personal experience, professional research, and coaching expertise, Arjun specializes in sustainable solutions that integrate full-body workouts, proper nutrition, and mindset shifts for long-term results.

In his debut book, "Flatten Your Belly," Arjun provides a step-by-step guide for men to achieve lasting belly-fat reduction. The book combines effective exercises, tailored dietary advice, and actionable tips to tackle challenges like stress and plateaus.

Arjun's relatable tone and encouraging approach empower readers to embrace a healthier, more energetic lifestyle. "Flatten Your Belly" is more than a fitness guide—it's a roadmap to lasting health, written by someone who shares your journey.

Acknowledgements

I owe my deepest gratitude to my parents, whose love, guidance, and support have shaped the foundation of my life and brought me into this beautiful world. Their unwavering belief in me has been my greatest source of strength.

I extend heartfelt thanks to my beloved spouse, Hemlata, whose encouragement and patience have been my anchor throughout this creative journey. To my sons, Mukul and Mehul, and my daughter, Riya, I am profoundly grateful for their inspiration, assistance, and shared enthusiasm, which played a vital role in crafting the content of this book. Your insights and love have been invaluable in bringing this project to life.

Above all, I bow in reverence to my Master, whose wisdom and guidance have brought purpose and meaning to my life. Without the light of your teachings, this endeavor would not have been possible.

Last but not the least, I must thank the Global humanitarian Organization, The Art of Living which really taught me how to live a Healthy Life and what is meaning of a Healthy Life.

This book is a tribute to all of you—a reflection of the love, strength, and wisdom you have bestowed upon me. Thank you for being an integral part of this journey.

Table of Contents

Contents

Flatten Your Belly, Transform Your Life: The Proven Blueprint for Men to Lose Belly Fat Fast"

- This title promises a transformation, not just in body shape but in overall life, appealing to men who want lasting change.

Introduction: Your Journey Starts Here

- **Overview of the Problem**: **Common Struggles Men Face with Belly Fat**

- In **"Flatten Your Belly, Transform Your Life: The Proven Blueprint for Men to Lose Belly Fat Fast"**, it's essential to first address the challenges men face when it comes to belly fat reduction. Men are often frustrated with their inability to shed those stubborn inches around the waist, despite their best efforts. These struggles stem from a combination of **lifestyle**, **genetics**, and **emotional factors**, all of which play a critical role in why belly fat accumulates and remains difficult to lose. Let's take a deeper look at each of these aspects.

- **1. Lifestyle: The Modern Challenge of Sedentary Living**

  Today's fast-paced world often leaves men with little time or energy to prioritize their health, leading to unhealthy lifestyle habits that contribute directly to belly fat accumulation.

  Poor Diet Choices: Many men consume high-calorie, low-nutrient foods, often opting for fast food, processed snacks, and sugary drinks due to convenience and stress. These poor dietary choices not only contribute to weight gain but also lead to insulin resistance, a key factor in belly fat storage.

Lack of Physical Activity: Sedentary jobs and long hours in front of screens contribute to a lack of physical activity, slowing down metabolism and reducing the body's ability to burn fat. Even with regular exercise, without the right combination of strength training, cardiovascular exercise, and recovery, belly fat can remain stubborn.

Busy Work and Family Life: As men juggle demanding careers, family obligations, and personal responsibilities, fitness often takes a backseat. Skipping workouts, poor sleep, and eating on the go contribute to unhealthy weight gain, particularly around the belly.

- **2. Genetics: The Unchangeable Factor**

Genetics play a significant role in determining where and how our bodies store fat. While we can't change our genes, understanding their impact can help men target belly fat more effectively.

Visceral Fat vs. Subcutaneous Fat: Men are genetically predisposed to store more **visceral fat**—the dangerous fat that surrounds internal organs—around their belly area. This type of fat is more challenging to lose and has a greater impact on health than subcutaneous fat (the fat under the skin).

Testosterone Levels: Testosterone, the hormone responsible for muscle mass and fat distribution in men, decreases with age, especially after 30. As testosterone levels drop, men tend to accumulate more fat around their abdomen and experience muscle loss, making fat loss even more difficult.

Fat Distribution: Some men are naturally more prone to storing fat around their belly due to their genetic make-up. While this might feel like an uphill battle, understanding this predisposition helps frame realistic goals and expectations, empowering men to work with their bodies rather than fight against them.

- **3. Emotional Factors: The Mental Barrier**

One of the most overlooked factors in belly fat loss is the psychological and emotional aspects that contribute to weight gain and make fat loss seem daunting.

Stress and Cortisol: Chronic stress is a significant contributor to belly fat. Stress triggers the release of **cortisol**, a hormone that not only increases appetite but also promotes fat storage in the abdominal area. Many men cope with stress by turning to comfort foods or skipping workouts, perpetuating the cycle of weight gain.

Body Image Issues: While women are often the focus of body image discussions, many men also struggle with how they perceive their bodies. A negative self-image or feeling inadequate can lead to emotional eating, poor lifestyle choices, and avoidance of fitness routines due to lack of motivation or confidence.

Emotional Eating and Cravings: Many men struggle with eating for emotional reasons—whether it's stress, boredom, or a desire for comfort. This form of emotional eating often leads to an overconsumption of calories, especially from sugar and processed foods, making it much harder to lose belly fat.

Motivational Barriers: Even when men know what they should be doing to lose belly fat, emotional barriers such as lack of motivation, fear of failure, or past weight loss setbacks can hinder their progress. The journey to flattening the belly is often psychological as much as it is physical.

In **"Flatten Your Belly, Transform Your Life,"** understanding these **lifestyle**, **genetic**, and **emotional factors** is the first step toward achieving lasting success. This book doesn't just focus on physical exercise and diet—it addresses the root causes of belly fat and provides a holistic, realistic approach to fat loss that empowers men to overcome the challenges in their lives. By acknowledging the real struggles men face, we can work together to create a strategy that tackles belly fat from every angle, making it possible to flatten the belly and transform your life for good.

The Promise: Outline the main goal of the book: helping men lose belly fat effectively, quickly, and sustainably.

How to Use This Book: A brief guide on how to navigate the chapters, encouraging readers to take action and follow the plan.

Chapter 1: The Hidden Dangers of Belly Fat

- **Why belly fat is more than just a cosmetic issue (health risks like heart disease, diabetes, etc.)**

In **"Flatten Your Belly, Transform Your Life: The Proven Blueprint for Men to Lose Belly Fat Fast"**, it's important to emphasize that belly fat is not just a cosmetic concern. While many men may initially focus on reducing belly fat for aesthetic reasons, it's crucial to understand the significant **health risks** associated with excess abdominal fat. Belly fat, especially **visceral fat** (the fat that lies deep within the abdominal cavity), poses serious health threats that extend far beyond appearances. This chapter will help men realize that losing belly fat is not just about looking better—it's about **living a longer, healthier life**.

1. Heart Disease: The Leading Cause of Death

Excess belly fat is a major contributor to **cardiovascular disease**, which is the leading cause of death for men, particularly those over 40. Visceral fat, the type of fat most commonly stored in the abdominal area, is metabolically active and releases harmful substances that can affect your heart and blood vessels.

Increased Cholesterol and Triglycerides: Belly fat has been shown to contribute to higher levels of **LDL cholesterol** (the "bad" cholesterol) and **triglycerides** in the blood. Both of these are risk factors for **atherosclerosis**, a condition where plaque builds up in the arteries, narrowing them and potentially leading to heart attacks and strokes.

Higher Blood Pressure: The accumulation of belly fat is linked to **high blood pressure** (hypertension). Visceral fat produces chemicals that can make blood vessels constrict, leading to higher blood pressure. Chronic hypertension increases the strain on the heart, leading to heart disease, heart failure, and even sudden cardiac arrest.

Inflammation: Visceral fat releases pro-inflammatory molecules called **cytokines**. This chronic low-grade inflammation can damage blood vessels and increase the likelihood of **atherosclerosis**, significantly raising the risk of heart disease.

2. Type 2 Diabetes: The Silent Epidemic

Excess belly fat is one of the key contributors to **insulin resistance**, which is the precursor to **type 2 diabetes**. Insulin resistance occurs when the body's cells no longer respond to insulin effectively, leading to high blood sugar levels.

Insulin Resistance: Fat stored around the abdomen (especially visceral fat) interferes with insulin's ability to regulate blood sugar. Over time, this resistance can lead to type 2 diabetes, a chronic condition that increases the risk of heart disease, kidney failure, nerve damage, and even amputations.

Increased Blood Sugar: When your body becomes resistant to insulin, your blood sugar levels rise, which can lead to **hyperglycaemia** (high blood sugar). This contributes to a higher risk of developing type 2 diabetes. Studies show that people with higher levels of abdominal fat are significantly more likely to develop insulin resistance than those with lower belly fat.

Metabolic Syndrome: Abdominal obesity is a key component of **metabolic syndrome**, a cluster of conditions—including high blood pressure, high blood sugar, high cholesterol, and excess belly fat—that increase the risk of heart disease, stroke, and diabetes. The more visceral fat you carry, the more likely you are to develop metabolic syndrome.

3. Increased Risk of Certain Cancers

Research has shown that excessive belly fat is linked to an increased risk of various cancers, making it a silent contributor to serious health issues.

Colorectal Cancer: Studies have shown that visceral fat increases the risk of colorectal cancer. The inflammatory markers released by visceral fat can encourage the growth of cancerous cells in the colon and rectum.

Liver Cancer: Excess abdominal fat is also associated with **non-alcoholic fatty liver disease (NAFLD)**, a condition where fat accumulates in the liver without alcohol consumption. NAFLD can progress to cirrhosis and liver cancer.

Prostate Cancer: Men with larger amounts of belly fat have a higher risk of developing aggressive forms of prostate cancer, possibly due to the inflammatory factors and hormones released by visceral fat.

Breast Cancer (in Men): Though rarer in men, **breast cancer** is still a concern, and studies suggest that higher belly fat can increase the risk of this cancer due to hormonal imbalances caused by excess fat.

4. Sleep Apnea and Respiratory Issues

Belly fat can contribute to **sleep apnea**, a condition in which breathing repeatedly stops and starts during sleep. This happens because excess fat in the abdomen can push up against the diaphragm and lungs, restricting airflow and leading to episodes of waking up gasping for air.

Obstructive Sleep Apnea: Men with excess belly fat are more likely to suffer from obstructive sleep apnea, which disrupts sleep patterns and leads to poor-quality rest. This not only causes daytime fatigue but also increases the risk of high blood pressure, heart disease, stroke, and diabetes.

Decreased Oxygen Intake: Excess fat around the belly can compress the chest cavity and reduce lung volume, making it harder to breathe and leading to reduced oxygen intake during sleep. This can also contribute to chronic fatigue and decrease overall energy levels.

5. Joint Pain and Mobility Issues

Carrying excess weight around the belly doesn't just affect internal organs—it also puts a strain on the skeletal system. The extra pounds can lead to inflammation in the joints, particularly in the knees and lower back, causing chronic pain and mobility issues.

Osteoarthritis: Abdominal obesity is associated with a higher risk of **osteoarthritis**, particularly in the knees. The added weight can cause wear and tear on the cartilage, leading to pain, stiffness, and difficulty moving.

Spinal Health: Belly fat can also impact the spine. The extra weight pulls on the lower back and leads to poor posture, which can result in back pain, herniated discs, and other spinal issues.

6. Mental Health Issues

The impact of belly fat extends beyond physical health—it also affects mental well-being. The frustration of being unable to lose belly fat can lead to feelings of helplessness, low self-esteem, and even depression.

- **Depression**: Studies have shown that individuals with higher levels of abdominal fat are more likely to experience **depression** and anxiety. This may be due to the physical discomfort caused by excess weight or the negative self-image associated with carrying extra pounds.

- **Stress and Anxiety**: The emotional toll of carrying belly fat, along with the physical symptoms of metabolic imbalance, can also trigger chronic stress and anxiety, further exacerbating the problem.

Conclusion: Why Losing Belly Fat is a Health Priority

Belly fat is not just about aesthetics—it's about protecting your long-term health. In **"Flatten Your Belly, Transform Your Life"**, we'll explore how reducing belly fat can significantly decrease your risk of heart disease, diabetes, and other chronic illnesses while also improving your mental health, energy, and quality of life. By understanding the deep-rooted health risks associated with excess abdominal fat, you'll be motivated to take the steps needed to transform your body—and your life.

- **The science behind visceral fat vs. subcutaneous fat.**

Why is Visceral Fat More Dangerous Than Subcutaneous Fat?

While both visceral and subcutaneous fat can contribute to weight gain and body composition issues, **visceral fat** poses far greater health risks. Here's why:

- **Metabolic Activity**: Visceral fat is far more active in terms of metabolism than subcutaneous fat. It secretes inflammatory cytokines and free-fatty acids directly into the bloodstream, which have a profound effect on your body's internal organs, hormones, and overall health.

- **Impact on Internal Organs**: Visceral fat surrounds and infiltrates vital organs such as the liver, pancreas, and intestines, directly affecting their function. Subcutaneous fat, while uncomfortable and unsightly, does not have the same direct impact on internal organs.

- **Heart Disease**: One of the most dangerous consequences of visceral fat is its contribution to heart disease. The fatty acids released by visceral fat can enter the liver and be converted into harmful substances that raise cholesterol levels, increase blood pressure, and promote atherosclerosis, all of which are major risk factors for heart disease.

- **Diabetes and Insulin Resistance**: The metabolic disruption caused by visceral fat leads to **insulin resistance**, which is a key factor in the development of type 2 diabetes. Insulin resistance is also linked to high blood sugar, high cholesterol, and high blood pressure, all of which increase the risk of heart disease.

- **Cancer and Chronic Illness**: The inflammation caused by visceral fat is not just limited to metabolic conditions; it also creates an environment that promotes the growth of cancerous cells. Studies have shown a clear link between high levels of visceral fat and an increased risk of developing certain types of cancer.

How to Target Visceral Fat

The good news is that visceral fat can be **reduced** with the right combination of diet, exercise, and lifestyle changes. Unlike subcutaneous fat, which is more easily lost through general weight loss, visceral fat requires targeted strategies to tackle effectively. Here are the best ways to reduce visceral fat:

1. **Dietary Changes**: Focus on a diet that is low in processed sugars, refined carbs, and unhealthy fats. Prioritize whole foods like vegetables, lean proteins, healthy fats (like omega-3s), and high-fiber foods, which help regulate blood sugar levels and reduce inflammation.

2. **Exercise**: Regular physical activity is crucial for reducing visceral fat. Cardiovascular exercises (like running,

swimming, or cycling) are particularly effective, but combining them with **strength training** can further accelerate fat loss by increasing muscle mass and boosting metabolism. High-intensity interval training (HIIT) is especially effective for targeting visceral fat.

3. **Stress Reduction**: Since stress leads to increased cortisol production, which promotes visceral fat storage, managing stress through activities like meditation, deep breathing exercises, or yoga can help lower visceral fat levels.

4. **Quality Sleep**: Aim for 7–9 hours of quality sleep per night. Poor sleep is linked to increased visceral fat accumulation, so establishing good sleep habits is crucial for fat loss.

Conclusion

Understanding the science behind **visceral** and **subcutaneous fat** is essential for anyone looking to improve their health and lose belly fat. While subcutaneous fat is more visible and easier to target, visceral fat is far more dangerous due to its effects on internal organs, metabolism, and overall health. By focusing on reducing visceral fat through a healthy diet, regular exercise, and stress management, you can significantly improve your health, lower your risk of chronic diseases, and transform your life. In **"Flatten Your Belly, Transform Your Life,"** we will show you how to take action against visceral fat and reclaim your health.

Chapter 2: The Male Body and Fat Storage

How Men Store Fat Differently: Testosterone, Genetics, and Metabolism

- Understanding how men store fat differently is crucial when it comes to developing an effective strategy for fat loss. Men's bodies tend to store fat in different areas and in different ways compared to women, largely due to a combination of **hormonal influences**, **genetics**, and **metabolism**. These factors help explain why men often accumulate fat around their belly and why their approach to fat loss requires specific attention.
- **Testosterone Levels and Fat Storage**
- One of the most significant factors influencing how men store fat is **testosterone**, the primary male sex hormone. Testosterone plays a key role in regulating body fat distribution, muscle mass, and overall metabolism.
- In general, men tend to store fat in the **abdominal area**, creating what is often referred to as a "beer belly" or **visceral fat**. This is because testosterone promotes fat storage around the midsection rather than in the hips or thighs. Lower testosterone levels, which can occur with age or due to lifestyle factors, tend to exacerbate belly fat accumulation. As men age, testosterone levels naturally decline, which can lead to an increase in abdominal fat, a decrease in muscle mass, and a slower metabolism. This is one reason why many men experience more difficulty losing belly fat as they grow older.
- **Genetics and Fat Distribution**
- Genetics also plays a significant role in fat storage patterns. Each person's genetic makeup influences where they store fat, how much fat they store, and how easily they can lose it. For men, genetics can determine

whether they are more likely to store fat in the belly (visceral fat) or around the thighs and arms (subcutaneous fat). Those with a genetic predisposition to store more fat around the midsection are at higher risk of developing **health complications** associated with visceral fat, such as heart disease and type 2 diabetes.

- Moreover, certain genetic factors can affect how efficiently your body burns fat. Some people are naturally predisposed to a higher resting metabolic rate, which allows them to burn fat more quickly, while others may have a slower metabolism that makes fat loss more challenging.
- **Metabolism and Fat Storage**
- Metabolism is the process by which your body converts food into energy. Men typically have a **higher metabolic rate** than women, largely because they tend to have more muscle mass. Muscle tissue burns more calories at rest than fat tissue, which gives men an advantage in terms of calorie expenditure. However, as men age and their testosterone levels decline, they may lose muscle mass and experience a corresponding slowdown in metabolism, making it harder to burn fat.
- In addition, certain metabolic factors—such as insulin resistance or an imbalance in hunger-regulating hormones—can contribute to fat storage. For men, elevated insulin levels, which often result from a diet high in refined sugars and processed foods, can trigger the body to store excess fat, particularly in the abdominal area.
- **Conclusion**
- In summary, men's fat storage patterns are shaped by a combination of **testosterone levels**, **genetic predisposition**, and **metabolic rate**. The hormonal effects of testosterone encourage the storage of fat around the abdomen, making it a challenge for men to

lose belly fat, especially as they age. Understanding these factors is critical when designing a fat-loss strategy. By addressing testosterone levels, optimizing metabolism through exercise and diet, and taking genetics into account, men can create a more targeted and effective approach to reducing belly fat and improving their overall health.

1.   Why belly fat is harder to lose for men and how to outsmart these biological factors.

Chapter 3: The Metabolism Factor – Why You Can't Ignore It

1.   What Is Metabolism and Why Is It Crucial for Fat Loss?

Metabolism refers to the complex biochemical processes that occur within your body to maintain life. It's how your body converts the food and drinks you consume into energy. This energy fuels essential functions such as breathing, circulating blood, repairing cells, and even thinking. Your metabolism operates 24/7, even when you're at rest.

At its core, metabolism can be broken into two main components: catabolism (breaking down molecules to release energy) and anabolism (building and storing energy). The total energy your body uses daily is known as your Total Daily Energy Expenditure (TDEE), which includes:

Basal Metabolic Rate (BMR): Energy used for basic body functions.

Thermic Effect of Food (TEF): Energy used to digest and process food.

Physical Activity: Energy used during exercise and non-exercise movements (e.g., fidgeting).

Why Is Metabolism Crucial for Fat Loss?

Metabolism is the foundation of fat loss because it dictates how efficiently your body burns calories. To lose fat, you need to create a calorie deficit—burning more calories than you consume. Here's how metabolism plays a role:

Resting Energy Burn: Your BMR accounts for 60-75% of daily calorie use. A higher BMR means your body burns more calories even at rest, which aids fat loss.

Exercise Impact: Physical activity increases calorie burn, but the degree depends on the efficiency of your metabolism. Regular exercise can boost your metabolism over time by increasing muscle mass, which burns more calories than fat at rest.

Diet and Metabolism: The foods you eat affect your metabolic rate. For instance, protein has a high thermic effect, meaning your body uses more energy to digest it compared to fats or carbohydrates.

Adaptation to Deficits: Prolonged calorie restriction can lead to metabolic adaptation, where your body slows its metabolism to conserve energy. Balancing deficits with occasional increases in calorie intake or resistance training can help mitigate this effect.

Optimizing Your Metabolism for Fat Loss

Build Muscle: Strength training increases muscle mass, boosting your BMR.

Stay Active: Incorporate both structured exercise and non-exercise activities.

Eat Smart: Focus on nutrient-dense foods, prioritize protein, and avoid severe calorie restriction.

Sleep and Stress Management: Poor sleep and chronic stress can disrupt hormonal balance, slowing your metabolism.

Understanding and optimizing your metabolism empowers you to approach fat loss more effectively. It's not just about eating less—it's about working with your body's natural processes to achieve sustainable results..

2. **How Slow Metabolism Affects Belly Fat and How to Rev It Up**

A sluggish metabolism can make losing belly fat feel like an uphill battle. Metabolism is your body's engine for burning calories and regulating energy. When it slows down, fewer calories are burned, and excess energy is more likely to be stored as fat—especially around the belly, which is particularly sensitive to hormonal and metabolic changes.

How Slow Metabolism Promotes Belly Fat

Calorie Surplus: A slow metabolism burns fewer calories, leading to a surplus even with moderate food intake. Excess calories are often stored as visceral fat, the deep belly fat surrounding organs.

Hormonal Impact: Slow metabolism can disrupt hormones like insulin and cortisol. Elevated cortisol levels, often linked to stress, promote fat storage in the abdominal region.

Reduced Fat Oxidation: A sluggish metabolic rate means your body is less efficient at breaking down fat for energy, making it harder to target belly fat.

How to Rev Up Your Metabolism

The good news is, you can take steps to boost your metabolism and reduce belly fat:

1. Build Muscle

Muscle tissue is metabolically active, burning more calories even at rest. Incorporate strength training exercises like squats, lunges, and deadlifts to increase muscle mass and fire up your metabolism.

2. Prioritize Protein

Protein-rich foods require more energy to digest and process, boosting your calorie burn. They also help preserve muscle mass during weight loss.

3. Stay Active

Increase your daily activity with high-intensity interval training (HIIT) or walking more throughout the day. Even small movements, like standing instead of sitting, can help.

4. Hydrate Well

Water is essential for metabolic processes. Drinking enough water can enhance your body's calorie-burning potential, especially before meals.

5. Manage Stress and Sleep

Chronic stress and poor sleep raise cortisol levels, slowing your metabolism and increasing belly fat storage. Prioritize 7-9 hours of quality sleep and practice stress management techniques like meditation or yoga.

6. Add Spices

Certain foods, like chili peppers, contain compounds (e.g., capsaicin) that temporarily boost metabolism.

Green tea and coffee, in moderation, can also provide a metabolic lift.

The Bottom Line

While a slow metabolism can make losing belly fat challenging, it's not an insurmountable obstacle. By adopting metabolism-boosting habits, you can enhance your body's calorie-burning power, target stubborn belly fat, and improve your overall health.

Chapter 4: Setting the Right Mindset for Success

1. **The Importance of Mental Focus and Motivation in Fat Loss**

   Fat loss is not just a physical challenge—it's a mental game. While diet and exercise are critical, mental focus and motivation are often the linchpins for sustained success. Science consistently highlights how mindset and psychological resilience influence the effectiveness and longevity of fat-loss efforts.

   How Mental Focus Affects Fat Loss

   I. **Self-Discipline and Habit Formation:**

   Mental focus enables you to stick to your calorie targets, prioritize healthy meals, and maintain a consistent workout schedule. A study in *Psychological Science* found that self-control and habit formation are essential for achieving weight-loss goals, particularly in environments full of temptations.

   II. **Mindful Eating:**
   Focused eating helps you recognize hunger and fullness cues, preventing overeating. Research published in *Appetite* shows that mindful eating can significantly reduce calorie intake and improve the quality of food choices.

   III. **Stress Management:**
   Mental focus helps manage stress, a common trigger for emotional eating and fat storage due to elevated cortisol levels. Regular mindfulness practices have been

proven to reduce stress-related eating behaviours and support fat loss.

Why Motivation Matters

I.   Sustaining Effort:

Motivation provides the drive to initiate and sustain fat-loss efforts. According to the *Journal of Obesity*, intrinsic motivation—focusing on personal health and well-being—is more effective than extrinsic motivators like appearance.

2. Overcoming Setbacks:

Fat loss is rarely linear, and motivation helps you bounce back from plateaus or slip-ups. A growth mindset, highlighted in *Mindset: The New Psychology of Success* by Dr. Carol Dweck, can foster resilience and long-term adherence.

3. Goal Setting and Achievement:

Motivation fuels goal setting, which has been linked to improved fat-loss outcomes. Studies show that SMART goals (Specific, Measurable, Achievable, Relevant, Time-bound) enhance motivation and keep you on track.

Strategies to Boost Mental Focus and Motivation

Set Clear, Meaningful Goals: Focus on achievable milestones tied to personal values, such as improved health or energy levels.

Track Progress: Use journals or apps to monitor your food intake, workouts, and body changes. Seeing progress reinforces motivation.

Visualize Success: Regularly picture yourself achieving your goals to strengthen commitment and focus.

Find Your "Why": Identify deep, personal reasons for fat loss beyond surface-level desires. This intrinsic motivation sustains long-term effort.

Celebrate Small Wins: Recognize progress, even small victories, to maintain momentum.

The Bottom Line

Mental focus and motivation are as crucial as diet and exercise in achieving fat-loss success. By cultivating self-discipline, managing stress, and setting meaningful goals, you can strengthen your mental resolve and create sustainable habits that lead to lasting results. Remember, a strong mind fuels a strong body.

2. **Creating a Sustainable Mindset Shift to Prioritize Health**

Sustainable health is more than a diet or workout routine—it starts with a mindset shift. Adopting long-term habits requires focusing on health as a lifestyle, not a temporary fix. Science highlights that changing how we think about health is key to creating lasting, positive behaviours.

Why Mindset Matters

I. **Growth Over Perfection:**
A growth mindset, as described by Dr. Carol Dweck, emphasizes learning and improvement rather than avoiding failure. This approach helps you bounce back from setbacks, whether it's missing a workout or

indulging in a high-calorie meal, without abandoning your goals.

II.   **Identity-Based Habits:**
Behavioural science research, including studies by Dr. James Clear (*Atomic Habits*), shows that sustainable change occurs when habits align with your identity. For example, instead of thinking, "I need to exercise," shifting to "I am someone who values fitness" fosters consistency.

III.   **Intrinsic Motivation:**
Sustainable health prioritizes intrinsic motivation—values like longevity, energy, and emotional well-being—over extrinsic factors like appearance. Studies in the *Journal of Health Psychology* highlight that focusing on internal benefits improves adherence to healthy behaviours.

Steps to Shift Your Mindset

Set Realistic, Meaningful Goals:

Break goals into achievable milestones tied to personal values, like improving energy or reducing stress, rather than focusing solely on weight loss.

Focus on the Process, Not the Outcome:

Instead of fixating on results, celebrate consistent actions—like cooking more meals at home or staying active daily. This process-oriented mindset fosters long-term commitment.

Embrace Flexibility:

Health is not about rigid routines. Studies in *Obesity Research* emphasize that flexible dieting and exercise approaches reduce burnout and improve adherence over time.

Practice Gratitude and Positivity:

Research in *Positive Psychology* links gratitude with healthier lifestyle choices. Acknowledge progress and focus on what your body can do, rather than criticizing imperfections.

Reframe Setbacks:

See challenges as learning opportunities, not failures. This resilience builds confidence in your ability to navigate obstacles.

Building Lasting Habits
Consistency Trumps Perfection: Aim for 80/20 adherence—be consistent most of the time while allowing for occasional indulgences.
Surround Yourself with Support: Community and accountability improve motivation. Share your goals with like-minded friends or join wellness groups.
Continue Learning: Educate yourself about nutrition, movement, and mental well-being to stay engaged and empowered.
The Bottom Line:
Shifting your mindset to prioritize health is about embracing growth, focusing on sustainable habits, and finding joy in the process. By reframing health as a lifelong journey, you can build a lifestyle that supports both your physical and mental well-being for years to come.

3. How to stay committed through challenges.

Chapter 5: Nutrition Hacks to Burn Belly Fat Fast

1. **The Critical Role of Diet in Belly Fat Reduction**

Diet plays a pivotal role in reducing belly fat, which is linked to serious health risks such as heart disease and diabetes. Scientific evidence highlights that targeted nutritional strategies can effectively combat visceral fat, the deep belly fat surrounding vital organs.

Key Dietary Strategies

Calorie Control:

A calorie deficit—burning more calories than consumed—is essential for fat loss. Research in *The American Journal of Clinical Nutrition* shows that sustained calorie control reduces overall and abdominal fat.

Prioritize Protein:

Protein increases satiety, preserves muscle mass, and boosts metabolism. Studies suggest diets rich in lean protein can specifically target belly fat by enhancing fat oxidation and reducing hunger.

Limit Added Sugars and Refined Carbs:

Excess sugar and refined carbs spike insulin, promoting fat storage in the abdominal area. Replacing these with whole grains and low-glycemic foods stabilizes blood sugar and reduces visceral fat.

Incorporate Healthy Fats:

Monounsaturated fats (e.g., avocados, nuts) and omega-3s (e.g., fatty fish) reduce inflammation and improve fat distribution. A study in *Diabetes Care* found that diets high in healthy fats help reduce central obesity.

Boost Fiber Intake:

Soluble fiber from foods like vegetables, legumes, and oats slows digestion, curbs appetite, and targets belly fat. Research shows a strong link between higher fiber intake and lower visceral fat levels.

The Bottom Line

Diet is the foundation of belly fat reduction. By focusing on whole, nutrient-dense foods and managing calorie intake, you can effectively decrease abdominal fat and improve overall health. Small, sustainable changes in eating habits yield long-term benefits.

2.   **The Best Foods to Accelerate Fat Loss**

Fat loss isn't just about cutting calories—it's about choosing foods that boost metabolism, control hunger, and optimize fat burning. Scientifically, a diet rich in protein, fiber, and healthy fats is key to accelerating fat loss while preserving muscle.

1. Protein: The Fat-Loss Powerhouse

Protein increases satiety, preserves muscle mass, and has a high thermic effect, meaning your body burns more calories digesting it.

Best Sources: Lean meats (chicken, turkey), eggs, fish (salmon, tuna), Greek yogurt, and plant-based proteins like tofu and lentils.

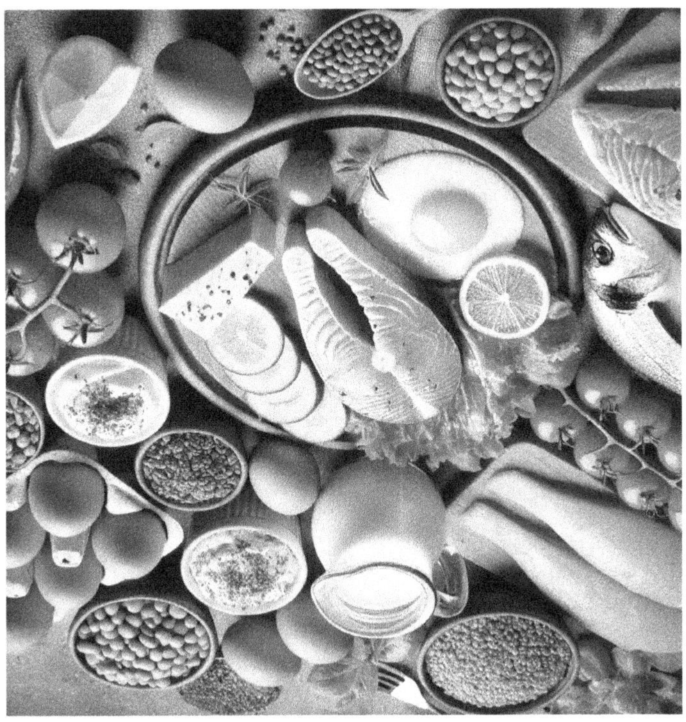

Why It Works: Studies show protein-rich diets enhance fat oxidation and reduce belly fat while maintaining lean body mass (*American Journal of Clinical Nutrition*).

2. Fiber: The Appetite Controller

Soluble fiber slows digestion, stabilizes blood sugar, and keeps you full longer, helping to curb overeating.

Best Sources: Oats, beans, lentils, flaxseeds, chia seeds, and non-starchy vegetables like broccoli and spinach.

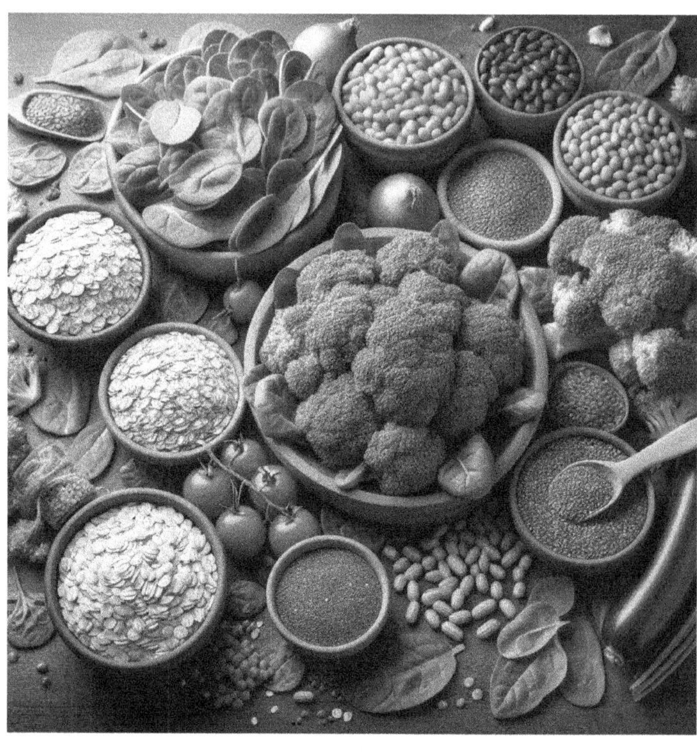

Why It Works: Research in *Obesity Reviews* links higher fiber intake with reduced body fat, particularly around the abdomen.

3. Healthy Fats: The Metabolism Boosters

Fats like omega-3s and monounsaturated fats reduce inflammation and improve fat metabolism. They also promote fullness, preventing calorie overconsumption.

Best Sources: Avocados, nuts (almonds, walnuts), seeds (chia, flax), olive oil, and fatty fish (salmon, mackerel).

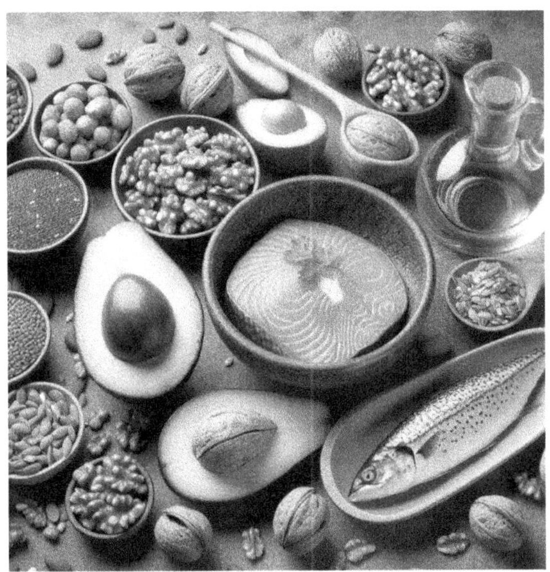

Why It Works: A study in *Diabetes Care* found that healthy fats, when replacing refined carbs, enhance fat loss and metabolic health.

The Bottom Line

Incorporating protein, fiber, and healthy fats into your diet not only accelerates fat loss but also supports overall health. Focus on nutrient-dense whole foods and balanced portions for sustainable results.

3. **The Worst Foods to Avoid for Fat Loss**

Certain foods can sabotage your fat-loss efforts by promoting fat storage, spiking blood sugar, and increasing hunger. Avoiding these "worst offenders" can help you stay on track and achieve sustainable results.

1. Sugary Drinks

Loaded with empty calories, sugary beverages like soda, sweetened teas, and energy drinks are a leading cause of weight gain.

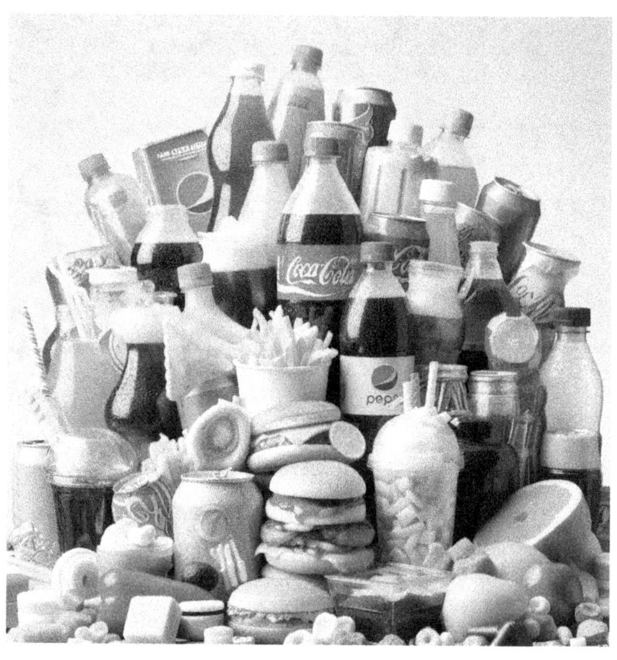

Why to Avoid: Studies in The American Journal of Clinical Nutrition show sugary drinks bypass satiety signals, leading to overconsumption and fat storage, especially in the belly area.

Better Alternative: Water, unsweetened tea, or sparkling water with a splash of citrus.

2. Processed Carbs

White bread, pastries, and other refined carbs cause rapid blood sugar spikes followed by crashes, leaving you hungry and prone to overeating.

Why to Avoid: Research links diets high in refined carbs to increased visceral fat and insulin resistance (*Journal of Nutrition*).

Better Alternative: Whole grains like quinoa, oats, and brown rice.

3. Trans Fats

Found in many fried foods, margarine, and packaged snacks, trans fats are artificial fats that promote inflammation and fat storage.

Why to Avoid: Studies in *Obesity Research* show trans fats increase abdominal fat and raise bad cholesterol levels.

Better Alternative: Healthy fats like olive oil, avocados, and nuts.

4. High-Calorie Processed Snacks

Chips, candy bars, and similar snacks combine high fat, sugar, and salt, triggering overeating without providing nutrients.

Why to Avoid: These hyper-palatable foods are engineered to override fullness cues, according to research in *Appetite*.

Better Alternative: Fresh fruit, nuts, or homemade snacks like air-popped popcorn.

The Bottom Line

Avoiding sugary drinks, refined carbs, trans fats, and processed snacks can significantly improve your fat-loss results. Focus on whole, nutrient-dense foods to support your health and weight-loss goals.

4. **Portion Control and Meal Timing: Keys to Fat Loss**

Effective fat loss isn't just about what you eat—it's also about how much and when you eat. Portion control and strategic meal timing, such as intermittent fasting and avoiding late-night eating, can enhance calorie management, metabolism, and fat-burning processes.

1. Portion Control

Eating large portions, even of healthy foods, can lead to calorie overconsumption.

Why It Works: Studies in The American Journal of Clinical Nutrition show that smaller portions reduce overall calorie intake without compromising satisfaction.

Tips: Use smaller plates, pre-portion snacks, and prioritize high-protein, high-fiber foods to feel full with fewer calories.

2. Intermittent Fasting (IF)

Intermittent fasting alternates periods of eating and fasting, such as the 16:8 method (16 hours of fasting, 8 hours of eating).

Why It Works: IF can improve insulin sensitivity and enhance fat oxidation, according to research in Cell Metabolism. It also reduces overall calorie intake naturally by limiting the eating window.

Tips: Start with a manageable fasting period, gradually extending as your body adapts.

3. Reducing Late-Night Eating

Late-night eating often leads to consuming high-calorie, low-nutrient foods and disrupts metabolic processes.

Why It Works: A study in *Nutrients* found that eating late increases fat storage and disrupts the body's circadian rhythm, impairing fat loss.

Tips: Set a "kitchen curfew," aiming to finish eating 2-3 hours before bedtime.

The Bottom Line

Portion control and meal timing, such as intermittent fasting and avoiding late-night meals, are powerful tools for optimizing fat loss. By managing portions and aligning meals with your body's natural rhythms, you can enhance results and build sustainable habits.

5. **Meal plans and grocery lists.**

Breakfast:

Scrambled eggs with spinach and avocado slices.

Whole-grain toast.

Lunch:

Grilled chicken salad with mixed greens, olive oil dressing, and quinoa.

Snack:

Greek yogurt with chia seeds and berries.

Dinner:

Baked salmon, steamed broccoli, and roasted sweet potatoes.

Optional Dessert:

Dark chocolate (70% cacao or higher).

Grocery List

Proteins: Chicken breast, salmon, eggs, Greek yogurt, tofu.

Whole Grains: Oats, quinoa, brown rice.

Fruits & Vegetables: Spinach, broccoli, berries, avocado, sweet potatoes.

Healthy Fats: Olive oil, nuts, seeds.

Extras: Green tea, dark chocolate, spices like turmeric and cinnamon.

The Bottom Line

A belly-fat-burning diet emphasizes protein, fiber, healthy fats, and whole foods while limiting processed and sugary options. Pair this meal plan with consistent activity and proper hydration for faster results!

Chapter 6: The Power of Strength Training for Belly Fat Loss

Why Strength Training is Essential for Men Over 30

Strength training is a critical tool for men over 30 aiming to lose belly fat and improve overall health. As metabolism slows with age and muscle mass naturally declines, targeted resistance exercises can counteract these changes and accelerate fat loss, especially around the abdomen.

The Science Behind Strength Training and Belly Fat

Preserves and Builds Muscle Mass

After 30, men lose about 3-5% of muscle mass per decade, which reduces calorie-burning capacity. Strength training preserves muscle and increases resting metabolic rate (RMR), helping to burn belly fat more efficiently.

Boosts Fat-Burning Hormones

Resistance training stimulates the release of testosterone and growth hormone, both of which decline with age and are crucial for fat metabolism. Research in *The Journal of Strength and Conditioning Research* shows that strength training enhances these hormones, reducing visceral fat.

Targets Belly Fat Specifically

While you can't spot-reduce fat, studies show that strength training reduces overall body fat, including dangerous visceral fat that accumulates around the belly. It also reshapes the body for a leaner appearance.

Effective Strength Training for Belly Fat

Compound Movements: Prioritize exercises like squats, deadlifts, bench presses, and rows to engage multiple muscle groups and maximize calorie burn.

High-Intensity Resistance Training (HIRT): Combine strength exercises with minimal rest to boost fat oxidation and metabolic rate post-workout.

Frequency: Aim for 3-4 sessions per week for optimal results.

The Bottom Line

Strength training is essential for men over 30 to combat age-related muscle loss, boost metabolism, and reduce belly fat. By incorporating regular resistance exercises, you'll improve body composition, enhance hormonal health, and achieve long-term fat-loss success.

1. **Key Exercises to Target Belly Fat: Full-Body Workouts and Core Strengthening**

Reducing belly fat is a common fitness goal, but it's important to note that spot-reduction is a myth. To effectively target belly fat, you need a combination of full-body workouts to burn calories and core-strengthening exercises to build muscle in your midsection. Here's a scientifically-backed guide:

1. Full-Body Workouts: The Foundation for Fat Loss

Full-body workouts are essential for burning calories and reducing overall body fat. When your body loses fat, your belly fat also decreases. Here are some of the most effective options:

High-Intensity Interval Training (HIIT):

HIIT involves short bursts of intense exercise followed by brief recovery periods. Studies show HIIT can reduce visceral fat (fat around the abdomen) more effectively than steady-state cardio. Example: 30 seconds of sprinting, followed by 60 seconds of walking, repeated for 15-20 minutes.

Strength Training:

Building muscle boosts your metabolism, leading to greater calorie burn at rest. Compound exercises like deadlifts, squats, and bench presses engage multiple muscle groups and torch calories. Example: Perform 3 sets of 10-12 reps for each major muscle group twice a week.

Cardio (Moderate to Vigorous Intensity):

Aerobic exercises like running, cycling, or swimming improve cardiovascular health and burn fat. Aim for at least 150 minutes of moderate or 75 minutes of vigorous activity weekly, as recommended by the WHO.

2. Core-Strengthening Exercises: Sculpt Your Midsection

While core exercises alone won't burn belly fat, they enhance muscle tone and improve posture, giving a leaner appearance. Key moves include:

Plank Variations:

Planks strengthen your entire core, including the deep abdominal muscles.
Try standard planks, side planks, or plank shoulder taps for 3 sets of 30-60 seconds.

Bicycle Crunches:

A study published in the *Journal of Strength and Conditioning Research* ranked this as one of the best abdominal exercises for activating the rectus abdominis.
Perform 3 sets of 15-20 reps per side.

Russian Twists:

This rotational exercise targets your obliques. Perform 3 sets of 20 twists (10 per side) using a weight or medicine ball for added intensity.

Mountain Climbers:

A dynamic, full-body exercise that engages your core and increases heart rate.
Perform for 30-60 seconds in 3 sets.

3. Combine with Proper Nutrition and Lifestyle

Exercise alone is not enough. Pair your workouts with a balanced diet rich in whole foods, lean proteins, healthy fats, and complex carbs. Additionally, prioritize sleep, as poor sleep can increase belly fat due to hormonal imbalances.

Takeaway

A holistic approach combining full-body workouts, core exercises, and a healthy lifestyle is the most effective way to reduce belly fat. Commit to consistency and challenge yourself progressively for the best results. Always consult a healthcare professional before starting a new fitness routine.

Weekly Workout Routine for Maximum Fat Burn: A Scientifically Proven Plan

Burning fat effectively requires a structured weekly workout routine that combines cardio, strength training, and recovery. By incorporating various exercise modalities, you can boost your metabolism, improve endurance, and maximize fat loss. Here's a proven weekly plan:

Day 1: High-Intensity Interval Training (HIIT)

Why it works: HIIT alternates short bursts of intense exercise with recovery periods, shown to burn more fat in less time than steady-state cardio.

1. **Workout Example:**
   1. Warm-up: 5 minutes (light jogging or dynamic stretches)
   2. HIIT Circuit:
      1. 30 seconds sprint, 1-minute walk (repeat for 20 minutes)
   3. Cool-down: 5 minutes of stretching

Day 2: Strength Training (Upper Body Focus)

Why it works: Strength training builds lean muscle, which increases resting metabolic rate (RMR), enhancing fat burn even when at rest.

1.   **Workout Example:** Perform 3 sets of 10-12 reps for each:

   1.   Push-ups or bench press

   2.   Bent-over rows

   3.   Shoulder presses

   4.   Tricep dips

   5.   Plank hold (30-60 seconds)

Day 3: Active Recovery or Yoga

Why it works: Recovery is vital for muscle repair and reducing cortisol levels, which can hinder fat loss. Yoga improves flexibility and reduces stress.

1.   **Workout Example:**

   1.   30–45 minutes of yoga or light activities like walking.

Day 4: Strength Training (Lower Body Focus)

Why it works: Large muscle groups in the lower body require more energy, leading to higher calorie burn during and after the workout.

1.   **Workout Example:** Perform 3 sets of 10-12 reps for each:

   1.   Squats (bodyweight or weighted)

   2.   Deadlifts

   3.   Lunges (per leg)

   4.   Step-ups

5.   Glute bridges

Day 5: Moderate-Intensity Cardio

Why it works: Sustained moderate cardio burns calories and improves cardiovascular endurance without overstraining the body.

1.   **Workout Example:**

    1.   30–45 minutes of jogging, cycling, or swimming at a steady pace.

Day 6: Full-Body Circuit Training

Why it works: Combining cardio and resistance training in a circuit maximizes calorie burn while building strength.

1.   **Workout Example:** Complete 3 rounds of the following, resting 1 minute between rounds:

    1.   Jump squats (15 reps)

    2.   Push-ups (15 reps)

    3.   Dumbbell rows (15 reps per arm)

    4.   Burpees (10 reps)

    5.   Mountain climbers (30 seconds)

Day 7: Rest or Active Recovery

Why it works: A rest day allows your body to repair and rebuild, critical for avoiding burnout and ensuring long-term fat loss.

1.   **Options:** Gentle stretching, foam rolling, or a light walk for 20–30 minutes.

Additional Tips for Success

1. **Nutrition:** Complement your workouts with a diet rich in lean proteins, healthy fats, whole grains, and plenty of vegetables.

2. **Hydration:** Drink enough water to stay energized and support metabolism.

3. **Sleep:** Aim for 7–9 hours of quality sleep nightly to optimize fat-burning hormones.

Takeaway

A well-rounded weekly routine combining HIIT, strength training, moderate cardio, and recovery is the most effective way to maximize fat burn. Stay consistent, track progress, and adjust intensity as needed to keep challenging your body.

Chapter 7: Cardiovascular Exercise for Burning Fat

How Cardio Helps Reduce Belly Fat: HIIT vs. Steady-State Cardio

Belly fat, particularly visceral fat, is linked to health risks like heart disease and diabetes. Cardio exercises are a scientifically proven way to target overall fat loss, including belly fat. By creating a calorie deficit and improving metabolic health, cardio plays a vital role in reducing abdominal fat. Here's how two popular forms of cardio—High-Intensity Interval Training (HIIT) and steady-state cardio—compare in their effectiveness.

The Science Behind Cardio and Belly Fat Loss

Caloric Burn: Cardio helps burn calories, promoting an energy deficit essential for fat loss.

Hormonal Effects: Regular cardio reduces insulin resistance and cortisol levels, which are associated with belly fat accumulation.

Metabolism Boost: Cardio, especially HIIT, elevates your metabolism for hours post-exercise, enhancing fat burning.

High-Intensity Interval Training (HIIT)

What it is: Alternating short bursts of intense effort with brief recovery periods.

Effectiveness on Belly Fat:

Studies show HIIT is particularly effective at reducing visceral fat, the dangerous fat stored around organs. HIIT stimulates the "afterburn effect" (excess post-exercise oxygen consumption, or EPOC), where your body continues burning calories post-workout.

Example HIIT Workout:

Warm-up: 5 minutes light jogging

Circuit:

30 seconds sprint

1-minute walk (repeat for 15–20 minutes)

Cool-down: 5 minutes stretching

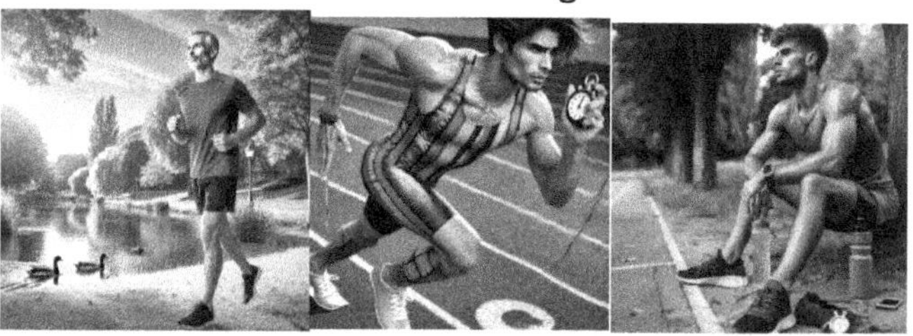

Advantages:

Time-efficient (shorter workouts with high impact)

Improves cardiovascular fitness and insulin sensitivity

Steady-State Cardio

What it is: Maintaining a consistent, moderate pace over a longer duration.

Effectiveness on Belly Fat:

While less intense than HIIT, steady-state cardio is effective for overall fat loss and improves endurance. It is particularly beneficial for beginners or those recovering from injuries. Consistent sessions can reduce subcutaneous fat (fat under the skin) and visceral fat when paired with a healthy diet.

Example Steady-State Workout:

30–60 minutes of jogging, cycling, or brisk walking at 60–70% of maximum heart rate.

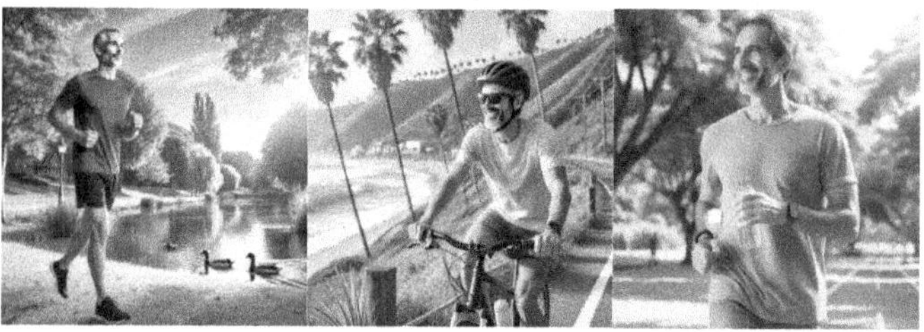

Advantages:
Easier to sustain over long periods
Lower impact, reducing injury risk

Which Is Better for Belly Fat Reduction?

HIIT: Best for those seeking quick results and higher calorie burn in shorter durations. It also promotes greater reductions in visceral fat, which is more metabolically active.

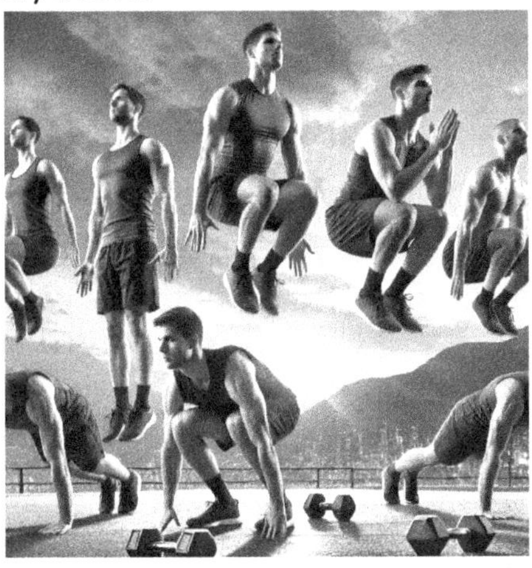

Steady-State Cardio: Ideal for beginners, those with joint concerns, or as a complement to strength training for overall fat loss.

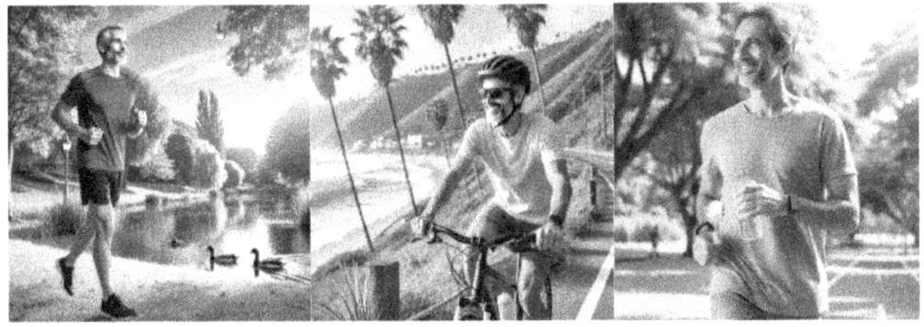

Combine Both for Maximum Results

A balanced routine incorporating both HIIT and steady-state cardio offers the best results for belly fat reduction. For example:

3 days of HIIT: Focus on high-intensity sessions to maximize fat burn and metabolic boost.

2–3 days of steady-state cardio: Use these as active recovery or longer endurance-building sessions.

Takeaway

Cardio, whether HIIT or steady-state, plays a crucial role in reducing belly fat by burning calories, improving metabolism, and enhancing overall health. Choose the type that suits your fitness level and preferences, or combine both for a comprehensive fat-loss strategy. Remember, cardio is most effective when paired with a balanced diet and strength training for long-term results.

Best Types of Cardio for Men: Running, Cycling, and Swimming

Cardio exercises are essential for men aiming to improve heart health, burn fat, and enhance overall fitness. Among the many forms of cardio, running, cycling, and swimming stand out as top choices, each offering unique benefits. Here's a scientifically-backed look at how these cardio types can elevate your fitness routine.

1. Running: The Classic Calorie Burner
Why it's effective:

Running is one of the most accessible and efficient forms of cardio. It burns significant calories and strengthens the cardiovascular system.

Benefits for Men:

High calorie burn (approximately 600–900 calories/hour depending on speed and weight).

Improves endurance, lung capacity, and lower body strength.

Reduces visceral fat, the harmful fat stored around organs, according to studies.

Tips for Best Results:

Incorporate intervals (e.g., sprints) for added fat burn.

Choose proper footwear to reduce injury risk.

Ideal For: Men looking for a high-impact workout to improve stamina and burn fat quickly.

2. Cycling: Joint-Friendly Cardio

Why it's effective:

Cycling provides a low-impact alternative to running, making it easier on the joints while still delivering excellent cardiovascular benefits.

Benefits for Men:

Burns 400–750 calories/hour depending on intensity.

Builds strong leg muscles, particularly quads, hamstrings, and calves.

Enhances heart health and supports endurance sports performance.

Tips for Best Results:

Use a combination of steady rides and hill climbs for strength and endurance.

Proper bike fit is crucial to avoid strain or injury.

Ideal For: Men seeking a low-impact, outdoor-friendly cardio option or those recovering from joint issues.

3. Swimming: Full-Body Conditioning
Why it's effective:
Swimming is a full-body workout that combines cardio with resistance training, thanks to water's natural resistance.
Benefits for Men:
Burns 500–700 calories/hour, depending on stroke and intensity.
Strengthens upper body, core, and lower body simultaneously.
Improves lung capacity and is particularly beneficial for those with joint or back issues.
Tips for Best Results:
Mix strokes (freestyle, backstroke, breaststroke) to engage different muscle groups.
Incorporate interval sets for added intensity.
Ideal For: Men looking for a low-impact, total-body workout that builds endurance and strength.

How to Choose the Right Cardio
Your choice depends on your fitness goals, preferences, and physical condition:
For Weight Loss: Running and cycling (HIIT sessions) are the most effective calorie burners.
For Joint Health: Opt for swimming or cycling to minimize impact.
For Total-Body Fitness: Swimming offers unmatched full-body conditioning.

Combine for Maximum Benefits

A varied routine is best for maintaining motivation and targeting multiple fitness goals. Example weekly schedule:

2 Days of Running: Focus on intervals or long-distance runs.

2 Days of Cycling: Combine steady rides with hill climbs.

1 Day of Swimming: Include interval sets to enhance endurance.

Takeaway

Running, cycling, and swimming are top cardio options for men, each providing distinct advantages. Combining these activities can create a balanced routine that promotes fat loss, cardiovascular health, and muscle endurance. Choose what suits your body and goals, and enjoy the journey to improved fitness!

How to structure cardio sessions to maximize fat loss.

Chapter 8: The Role of Recovery: Sleep and Stress Management

1. **The Impact of Sleep and Stress on Belly Fat: A Scientific Perspective**

   Belly fat, particularly visceral fat, is not just a cosmetic concern—it poses significant health risks, including heart disease, diabetes, and inflammation. While diet and exercise are crucial for reducing belly fat, sleep and stress play equally vital roles. Here's how these factors influence fat accumulation and strategies to address them.

   The Role of Sleep in Belly Fat Reduction
   Why sleep matters:
   Sleep is essential for hormonal balance, metabolism, and overall health. Poor sleep quality or insufficient sleep is directly linked to increased belly fat due to disruptions in metabolic processes.
   Hormonal Effects:
   Increased Ghrelin: Lack of sleep boosts this "hunger hormone," leading to overeating.
   Decreased Leptin: Sleep deprivation reduces leptin, the hormone responsible for satiety.
   Elevated Cortisol: Poor sleep raises cortisol levels, a stress hormone linked to fat storage, particularly in the abdominal area.
   Metabolic Impact:
   Studies show that individuals sleeping fewer than 6 hours per night are more likely to accumulate visceral fat over time compared to those sleeping 7–9 hours.
   Actionable Tips for Better Sleep:
   Establish a consistent sleep schedule.

Avoid caffeine and electronic screens at least 2 hours before bedtime.

Create a sleep-friendly environment (cool, dark, and quiet).

How Stress Contributes to Belly Fat

Why stress matters:

Chronic stress triggers a cascade of physiological responses that promote belly fat storage.

The Cortisol Connection:

When stressed, the body releases cortisol, a hormone that increases appetite and encourages fat storage around the midsection.

Elevated cortisol also drives cravings for high-calorie, sugary foods, further contributing to weight gain.

Behavioural Impact of Stress:

Emotional eating: Stress often leads to overeating unhealthy comfort foods.

Reduced activity: Stress can decrease motivation to exercise, exacerbating fat accumulation.

Actionable Tips for Managing Stress:

Practice mindfulness techniques, such as meditation or deep breathing.

Engage in regular physical activity to reduce cortisol levels naturally.

Seek social support or consider therapy to address chronic stress.

The Sleep-Stress-Belly Fat Cycle

Poor sleep and chronic stress often reinforce each other, creating a vicious cycle:

Stress disrupts sleep, leading to hormonal imbalances that promote fat storage.

Lack of sleep amplifies stress, further elevating cortisol and hindering fat loss.
Breaking this cycle is essential for reducing belly fat effectively.

Key Strategies for Addressing Sleep and Stress
Prioritize Sleep Hygiene:
Ensure 7–9 hours of quality sleep per night to regulate appetite-controlling and stress hormones.
Incorporate Stress-Relief Practices:
Yoga, journaling, or spending time in nature can help reduce cortisol levels.
Adopt a Balanced Lifestyle:
Pair stress management and sleep hygiene with a healthy diet and regular exercise for optimal results.

Takeaway
Sleep and stress have a profound impact on belly fat. Insufficient sleep and chronic stress disrupt hormonal balance, driving fat storage in the abdominal region. Addressing these factors through lifestyle changes can significantly enhance your fat loss efforts, improve overall health, and lower your risk of chronic diseases.

2. **Strategies for Improving Sleep Quality and Reducing Stress: A Scientific Guide**
Sleep and stress are interconnected pillars of mental and physical well-being. Poor sleep quality can elevate stress levels, while chronic stress disrupts sleep patterns. This vicious cycle not only impacts daily performance but also increases the risk of health issues like obesity, heart disease, and weakened immunity. Here are scientifically proven strategies to enhance sleep and manage stress effectively.

1. Establish a Consistent Sleep Routine

Why it works:

The body's circadian rhythm, or internal clock, thrives on consistency. Irregular sleep schedules disrupt this rhythm, making it harder to fall and stay asleep.

How to do it:

Go to bed and wake up at the same time every day, even on weekends.

Create a relaxing bedtime routine, such as reading or meditating, to signal your body it's time to sleep.

2. Optimize Your Sleep Environment

Why it works:

External factors like noise, light, and temperature significantly influence sleep quality.

How to do it:

Keep your bedroom cool (60–67°F or 15–20°C) and dark. Use blackout curtains or an eye mask to block light. Reduce noise with earplugs or a white noise machine.

3. Limit Stimulants and Electronics Before Bed

Why it works:

Caffeine and blue light from screens interfere with melatonin production, the hormone responsible for sleep.

How to do it:

Avoid caffeine at least 6 hours before bedtime.

Stop using electronic devices (phones, laptops, TVs) 1–2 hours before sleep.

Use night mode on devices or blue light-blocking glasses if screen use is unavoidable.

4. Practice Relaxation Techniques for Stress Reduction

Why it works:

Relaxation exercises activate the parasympathetic nervous system, lowering stress hormones like cortisol.

How to do it:

Deep Breathing: Inhale deeply for 4 seconds, hold for 7 seconds, and exhale for 8 seconds. Repeat for 5 minutes.

Progressive Muscle Relaxation: Gradually tense and relax each muscle group, starting from your toes to your head.

Meditation or Mindfulness: Focus on the present moment using apps like Headspace or Calm for guided sessions.

5. Engage in Regular Physical Activity

Why it works:

Exercise helps reduce stress and improves sleep by regulating hormones and promoting deeper sleep cycles.

How to do it:

Aim for at least 30 minutes of moderate-intensity exercise most days.

Avoid vigorous exercise within 2–3 hours of bedtime, as it can disrupt sleep.

6. Adopt a Balanced Diet

Why it works:

Nutrition affects both stress levels and sleep quality. Certain foods promote relaxation, while others can trigger stress or disrupt sleep.

How to do it:

Include sleep-friendly foods like bananas, almonds, and fatty fish, which are rich in magnesium, tryptophan, or omega-3s.
Avoid heavy meals, alcohol, and sugary foods close to bedtime.

7. Manage Stress Through Cognitive Behavioural Techniques

Why it works:
Cognitive-behavioural therapy (CBT) helps reframe negative thought patterns, reducing stress and improving mental well-being.

How to do it:
Identify stress triggers and challenge irrational fears or worries.
Journaling: Write down concerns and potential solutions to release mental tension.

8. Seek Professional Help When Needed

Why it works:
Chronic sleep issues or unmanageable stress may require specialized intervention.

How to do it:
Consult a sleep specialist if you suspect disorders like insomnia or sleep apnea.
Seek therapy or counselling for long-term stress management.

Takeaway
Improving sleep quality and reducing stress requires a combination of lifestyle adjustments and mindfulness practices. By establishing consistent routines, optimizing your environment, and adopting relaxation

techniques, you can break the sleep-stress cycle and enhance overall well-being. Start small, stay consistent, and seek support when needed for lasting benefits.

Relaxation Techniques: Meditation and Deep Breathing for Stress Relief

Relaxation techniques like meditation and deep breathing are scientifically proven methods to reduce stress, promote mental clarity, and improve overall well-being. These practices activate the parasympathetic nervous system, the body's "rest and digest" mode, countering the effects of chronic stress. Here's a closer look at how they work and how to practice them.

1. Meditation: Cultivating Mindfulness and Calm

How It Works:

Meditation trains your mind to focus and be present, reducing overthinking and stress. It lowers levels of cortisol (the stress hormone) and enhances emotional resilience.

Scientific Benefits:

1. Improves focus and mental clarity by increasing gray matter in the brain.
2. Reduces symptoms of anxiety and depression, as shown in studies published in *JAMA Internal Medicine.*
3. Lowers blood pressure and enhances heart health.

How to Practice Meditation:

1. **Mindfulness Meditation:**
   1. Sit comfortably in a quiet space.
   2. Close your eyes and focus on your breath, sensations, or a mantra.

3. When your mind wanders, gently bring your attention back.
4. Start with 5–10 minutes daily and gradually increase.
2. **Guided Meditation:** Use apps like Headspace, Calm, or Insight Timer for structured sessions.

2. Deep Breathing: Restoring Balance and Calm

How It Works:

Deep breathing slows your heart rate, reduces blood pressure, and signals your brain to relax. This technique increases oxygen intake, improving focus and emotional regulation.

Scientific Benefits:

1. Reduces stress by lowering cortisol levels and promoting a calm state.
2. Enhances lung function and oxygen delivery to cells.
3. Boosts immunity by reducing inflammation caused by chronic stress.

How to Practice Deep Breathing:

1. **4-7-8 Breathing Technique:**
    1. Inhale deeply through your nose for 4 seconds.
    2. Hold your breath for 7 seconds.
    3. Exhale slowly through your mouth for 8 seconds.
    4. Repeat 4–8 cycles.
2. **Diaphragmatic Breathing (Belly Breathing):**
    1. Sit or lie down in a comfortable position.
    2. Place one hand on your chest and the other on your belly.

3.   Inhale deeply through your nose, allowing your belly to rise.
4.   Exhale fully, feeling your belly fall.
5.   Practice for 5–10 minutes daily.

Incorporating Relaxation Techniques into Daily Life

1.   **Start Small:** Dedicate 5–10 minutes daily to meditation or deep breathing.
2.   **Create a Routine:** Pair these practices with existing habits, like starting your day or winding down before sleep.
3.   **Be Consistent:** Regular practice yields long-term benefits.

Takeaway

Meditation and deep breathing are simple yet powerful techniques to manage stress, enhance focus, and improve overall health. With consistent practice, these methods can help you lead a calmer, more balanced life.

Chapter 9: Busting the Myths: Common Belly Fat Loss Mistakes

1. Addressing Common Myths About Fat Loss: Spot Reduction and Fast-Fix Supplements

The journey to fat loss is often clouded by misconceptions that can mislead efforts and waste time and money. Two of the most persistent myths are the ideas of spot reduction and the effectiveness of fast-fix supplements. Here's what science has to say about these claims.

Myth 1: Spot Reduction Works for Fat Loss

The Claim:

Performing targeted exercises (e.g., crunches) will burn fat in specific areas like the belly or thighs.

The Reality:

Spot reduction is a myth. Fat loss occurs systemically, meaning your body decides where fat is burned based on genetics, hormones, and overall activity level.

Scientific Evidence:

A 2013 study published in the *Journal of Strength and Conditioning Research* found that doing targeted abdominal exercises for six weeks did not significantly reduce abdominal fat. Instead, the body reduces fat evenly across different areas when a calorie deficit is achieved.

What Actually Works:

Calorie Deficit: Burn more calories than you consume through a combination of diet and full-body exercise.

Cardio and Strength Training: Combine high-intensity cardio (like HIIT) with strength training to maximize fat burning and muscle retention.

Myth 2: Fast-Fix Supplements Can Melt Fat

The Claim:

Supplements like "fat burners" or detox teas promise rapid fat loss without effort.

The Reality:

Most fat-loss supplements lack solid scientific backing. While some ingredients (like caffeine or green tea extract) may slightly boost metabolism, their effects are negligible without proper diet and exercise.

Scientific Evidence:

A 2012 review in *Obesity Reviews* concluded that many weight-loss supplements show only minimal effects, often not enough to justify their cost or potential side effects.

"Detox teas" and similar products often lead to temporary weight loss due to water loss, not fat reduction, and can disrupt metabolism if overused.

What Actually Works:

Whole Foods Diet: Focus on nutrient-dense, whole foods to support fat loss naturally.

Patience and Consistency: Sustainable fat loss comes from gradual lifestyle changes, not quick fixes.

Key Takeaways for Effective Fat Loss

Adopt a Holistic Approach: Fat loss is best achieved through a combination of a balanced diet, regular exercise, and proper sleep.

Ignore the Gimmicks: Avoid supplements or programs promising effortless, rapid results.

Be Consistent: Sustainable progress requires patience and commitment over time.

The Bottom Line

Spot reduction and fast-fix supplements are myths that distract from evidence-based approaches to fat loss. Focus on creating a calorie deficit through a balanced lifestyle, and trust the process for long-term, sustainable results.

How to Avoid Shortcuts That Sabotage Fat Loss Progress

Fat loss is a journey that requires consistency, patience, and evidence-based strategies. Shortcuts, though tempting, often undermine long-term success and lead to frustration. Here's how to identify and avoid common pitfalls while staying on track for sustainable fat loss.

1. Avoid Crash Diets

Why They Fail:

Crash diets promise rapid weight loss by severely restricting calories, but they often lead to muscle loss, slowed metabolism, and rebound weight gain.

The Science:

Studies in *The American Journal of Clinical Nutrition* show that extreme calorie deficits can lower resting metabolic rate, making it harder to sustain weight loss.

What to Do Instead:

1.   Aim for a moderate calorie deficit of 500–750 calories/day.

2.   Focus on nutrient-dense foods to stay full and energized.

2. Say No to Fat-Loss Supplements and Detox Products

Why They Fail:

Products like "fat burners" and detox teas often make exaggerated claims and may lead to side effects like dehydration, nutrient imbalances, or digestive issues.

The Science:

A 2012 review in *Obesity Reviews* found limited or negligible effects from most weight-loss supplements. Any initial weight loss is typically due to water loss, not fat.

What to Do Instead:

1.   Prioritize whole foods and a balanced diet.

2.   Let your liver and kidneys handle detoxification naturally—they're designed for it.

3. Don't Overdo Cardio or Skip Strength Training

Why It Fails:

Excessive cardio without strength training can lead to muscle loss, making it harder to maintain a healthy body composition.

The Science:

A study in *Obesity* found that combining strength training with cardio is more effective for fat loss while preserving lean muscle.

What to Do Instead:

1. Incorporate 2–3 days of strength training alongside cardio.

2. Focus on compound movements (e.g., squats, deadlifts) to target multiple muscle groups.

4. Avoid Unrealistic Expectations

Why They Fail:

Chasing quick results can lead to frustration and burnout. Sustainable fat loss is a slow process, with a typical healthy rate of 0.5–1 pound per week.

The Science:

Research in *The Journal of the Academy of Nutrition and Dietetics* highlights that gradual weight loss is more likely to be maintained long-term.

What to Do Instead:

1. Celebrate small victories, like consistent workouts or healthier meal choices.

2. Focus on long-term habits rather than short-term outcomes.

5. Ditch "All-Or-Nothing" Thinking

Why It Fails:

Perfectionism can lead to giving up after minor setbacks, like overeating or missing a workout.

The Science:

Behavioural studies suggest that self-compassion promotes resilience and helps people stay consistent with their goals.

What to Do Instead:

1. Accept that slip-ups are part of the process.

2. Get back on track with your next meal or workout instead of dwelling on the setback.

Sustainable Strategies for Fat Loss Success

1. **Focus on Consistency Over Perfection:** Small, consistent changes lead to long-term results.

2. **Choose a Holistic Approach:** Balance diet, exercise, sleep, and stress management.

3. **Trust the Process:** Avoid gimmicks and shortcuts that promise quick results.

The Bottom Line

Shortcuts might promise fast results, but they often sabotage your fat loss progress by causing muscle loss, metabolic slowdown, or unsustainable habits. Stick to evidence-based methods, embrace the journey, and prioritize long-term health for lasting success.

Chapter 10: How to Handle Plateaus and Stay Motivated

1. **Understanding Weight Loss Plateaus and How to Break Through Them**

Weight loss plateaus are a common hurdle in any fat-loss journey. After initial progress, the scale may stop moving despite consistent efforts. This plateau occurs when your body adapts to changes in diet and exercise. Understanding why plateaus happen and how to overcome them is key to maintaining momentum.

What Causes Weight Loss Plateaus?

Metabolic Adaptation:

As you lose weight, your metabolism slows down because a smaller body requires fewer calories to maintain itself. This phenomenon, known as adaptive thermogenesis, can stall weight loss.

Reduced Calorie Deficit:

Over time, what was once a calorie deficit becomes maintenance as your energy needs decrease.

Loss of Lean Muscle Mass:

If muscle mass decreases during weight loss, your resting metabolic rate (RMR) also declines, slowing fat loss.

Water Retention or Hormonal Fluctuations:

Factors like stress, sleep deprivation, or high sodium intake can lead to temporary water retention, masking fat loss.

How to Break Through a Weight Loss Plateau

Reassess Your Calorie Intake

Why it works: Your calorie needs change as you lose weight. Eating the same number of calories that initially created a deficit might now only maintain your weight.

What to do: Use a calorie calculator to adjust your intake based on your new weight and activity level.

Increase Physical Activity

Why it works: Adding exercise increases calorie expenditure and can help overcome a slowed metabolism.

What to do:

Add high-intensity interval training (HIIT) to your routine for a metabolic boost.

Increase non-exercise activity thermogenesis (NEAT), like walking or household chores.

Prioritize Strength Training

Why it works: Building muscle increases your RMR, allowing you to burn more calories at rest.

What to do: Focus on compound movements (e.g., squats, deadlifts) and train major muscle groups 2–3 times per week.

Mix Up Your Exercise Routine

Why it works: The body adapts to repetitive workouts, reducing their effectiveness.

What to do: Try new activities, increase intensity, or vary workout duration to challenge your body.

Focus on Sleep and Stress Management

Why it works: Poor sleep and chronic stress increase cortisol levels, which can hinder fat loss and promote fat storage.

What to do:

Aim for 7–9 hours of quality sleep.

Practice relaxation techniques like meditation or deep breathing.

Incorporate Diet Breaks or Refeeds

Why it works: Briefly increasing calorie intake can reset hormones like leptin, which regulate hunger and metabolism.

What to do:

Take a controlled diet break for 1–2 weeks, increasing calories to maintenance levels while eating healthy foods.

When to Seek Professional Help

If you've tried these strategies and still can't break through the plateau, consult a registered dietitian, trainer, or medical professional. They can assess underlying factors like hormonal imbalances or metabolic conditions.

Takeaway

Weight loss plateaus are a natural part of the process and a sign that your body is adapting. Breaking through requires a strategic approach—reassess your diet, mix up your workouts, and focus on overall lifestyle improvements. With patience and consistency, you can overcome plateaus and continue progressing toward your goals..

2. **How to Track Progress Beyond the Scale:**

Measurements and Body Composition

Relying solely on the scale to measure progress during a fitness journey can be misleading. Weight fluctuations often result from factors like water retention, muscle gain, or hormonal changes, not fat loss. Tracking other metrics such as body measurements and body composition provides a more accurate picture of your progress.

1. Use Body Measurements

Why it works:

Measuring specific areas of your body shows where changes are occurring, even if the scale doesn't move.

How to do it:

Tools: Use a flexible measuring tape.

Key Areas to Measure:

Waist: Measure just above the belly button.

Hips: Measure the widest part of your hips.

Chest: Measure across the fullest part.

Thighs, Arms: Measure around the thickest area.

Frequency: Track measurements once every 2–4 weeks for consistent results.

Scientific Insight:

Research shows that waist circumference is a better indicator of health improvements, particularly for cardiovascular risk, than scale weight alone.

2. Monitor Body Composition

Why it works:

Body composition distinguishes between fat mass and lean mass (muscles, bones, organs). Losing fat while gaining muscle may keep your weight steady but improve your overall fitness and health.

How to do it:

Bioelectrical Impedance Scales: Affordable and accessible but less precise.

Skinfold Calipers: Measure body fat percentage using pinch tests at specific body points.

DEXA Scans or Bod Pods: Offer highly accurate readings of fat and muscle distribution but may require professional facilities.

Scientific Insight:

A study in *Obesity* highlights that increased muscle mass improves metabolism, even if weight loss isn't dramatic.

3. Take Progress Photos

Why it works:

Visual evidence over time can highlight changes in muscle tone, posture, and fat loss that numbers might not reflect.

How to do it:

Wear similar clothing and use consistent lighting.

Take front, side, and back photos every 4–6 weeks.

4. Track Performance Improvements

Why it works:

Progress isn't just about appearance—it's also about how your body functions.

How to do it:

Log workout performance: Track increased weights, reps, or endurance during exercises.

Monitor energy levels and how you feel during daily activities.

Scientific Insight:

Strength and endurance improvements often precede visible changes, indicating better health and fitness.

5. Pay Attention to Non-Scale Victories (NSVs)

Why it works:

NSVs reflect overall lifestyle improvements, including better health and well-being.

Examples of NSVs:

Clothes fitting better.

Improved sleep quality.

Reduced stress levels.

Lower resting heart rate or improved blood pressure.

Takeaway

The scale is just one tool for tracking progress. By incorporating measurements, body composition analysis, photos, and performance tracking, you can gain a holistic understanding of your journey. Celebrate non-scale victories and remember that progress is about overall health, not just a number.

4. Maintaining Motivation When Results Seem Slow

Slow progress can be frustrating, but staying motivated is crucial for long-term success. Sustainable health and fitness changes take time, and even small steps lead to significant outcomes when compounded over weeks and months. Here are scientifically proven strategies to keep your motivation high during plateaus or slow progress.

1. Set Realistic and Specific Goals

Why it works:

Clear, attainable goals give you a sense of purpose and direction, reducing the risk of burnout.

How to do it:

Use SMART goals: Specific, Measurable, Achievable, Relevant, and Time-bound.

Example: "Lose 1 pound per week by tracking meals and exercising 4 times a week."

Scientific Insight:

Studies in *Psychological Bulletin* show that people with specific, incremental goals are more likely to stay committed.

2. Track Non-Scale Progress

Why it works:

Progress is more than a number on the scale. Tracking improvements in strength, endurance, energy levels, or clothing fit can boost motivation.

How to do it:

Log workout performance: Track heavier weights, faster run times, or increased stamina.

Celebrate non-scale victories like better sleep, reduced stress, or healthier food choices.

3. Focus on the Process, Not Just the Outcome

Why it works:

Enjoying daily habits, like cooking healthy meals or trying new exercises, creates intrinsic motivation.

How to do it:

Shift focus from "losing 10 pounds" to "staying active and eating nourishing foods."

Reward consistency, such as completing all workouts in a week, rather than short-term outcomes.

4. Practice Self-Compassion

Why it works:

Being kind to yourself reduces the likelihood of giving up after setbacks, fostering resilience.

How to do it:

Avoid negative self-talk like "I'm failing." Instead, reframe it: "Progress takes time, and I'm doing my best."

Treat slip-ups as learning opportunities rather than failures.

Scientific Insight:

A study in *Health Psychology* found that self-compassion helps people maintain healthy behaviors over time.

5. Find a Support System

Why it works:

Accountability and encouragement from others can keep you motivated when your own drive wanes.

How to do it:

Join a fitness class or online community.

Share your goals with a friend or hire a coach for guidance.

6. Reassess and Adjust Your Plan

Why it works:

Sometimes, slow progress indicates the need for change. Small adjustments can reignite your momentum.

How to do it:

Reevaluate your calorie intake, workout routine, or recovery strategies.

Incorporate variety, such as trying new exercises or meal ideas.

7. Visualize Your Long-Term Success

Why it works:

Imagining how you'll feel and look after achieving your goals reinforces your commitment.

How to do it:

Use visualization techniques to picture yourself stronger, healthier, and more confident.

Write down your "why"—the deeper reason you want to achieve your goal—and revisit it often.

Takeaway

Progress may be slow, but every effort brings you closer to your goal. Focus on building sustainable habits, celebrate small wins, and stay patient. With consistent effort and a positive mindset, success is inevitable.

Chapter 11: How Losing Belly Fat Can Transform Your Confidence and Energy

1.   The Psychological Benefits of Losing Belly Fat:

Improved Self-Esteem and Body Image

Losing belly fat is often pursued for physical health benefits, but its psychological advantages are equally significant. Achieving a healthier body composition can profoundly impact mental well-being, boosting self-esteem and improving body image. Here's how science explains these positive effects.

1. Enhanced Self-Esteem

Why It Happens:

Self-esteem is closely tied to body confidence. Losing belly fat often leads to improved fitness, better posture, and clothing fitting more comfortably, contributing to a sense of accomplishment.

Scientific Evidence:

A 2019 study in *Body Image* revealed that individuals who reduced body fat experienced greater self-confidence, regardless of their starting weight. Achieving health goals fosters a sense of control and pride, positively affecting self-esteem.

Practical Impact:

Increased motivation to maintain a healthier lifestyle.

Improved performance in social, professional, or personal interactions due to greater confidence.

2. Improved Body Image

Why It Happens:

Body image is influenced by how you perceive your appearance. Reducing belly fat can help align your physical state with your desired body image, creating a more positive self-perception.

Scientific Evidence:

A study in *The Journal of Behavioral Medicine* found that regular exercise, even without significant weight loss, improved body satisfaction. Combined with visible fat loss, the psychological benefits are even more pronounced.

Practical Impact:

Reduced body dissatisfaction, which is linked to lower rates of depression and anxiety.

Better relationships, as improved self-perception fosters confidence in social settings.

3. Stress and Anxiety Reduction

Why It Happens:

Abdominal fat is often linked to higher cortisol levels, the stress hormone. Losing belly fat through exercise and better nutrition can lower cortisol, reducing feelings of stress and anxiety.

Scientific Evidence:

A 2020 review in *Psychology Research and Behaviour Management* highlighted the mental health benefits of exercise-driven fat loss, including reduced stress and enhanced emotional regulation.

Practical Impact:

Greater ability to handle challenges calmly and effectively.

Improved focus and productivity due to lower anxiety levels.

4. Enhanced Mood and Mental Health

Why It Happens:

Fat loss efforts typically involve regular exercise and balanced nutrition, which are proven to improve mood and brain health. The process itself can create a sense of purpose and achievement.

Scientific Evidence:

A study in *The Lancet Psychiatry* found that physical activity improves mental well-being by increasing endorphins and reducing depressive symptoms.

Practical Impact:

Elevated mood, leading to a more optimistic outlook.

Better coping mechanisms for daily stressors.

Key Takeaways

Losing belly fat is more than a physical transformation—it can lead to significant psychological benefits, such as boosted self-esteem, improved body image, and reduced stress. By focusing on sustainable lifestyle changes, the mental health rewards can be as life-changing as the physical ones. Celebrate each milestone, and remember that progress is about feeling better inside and out.

2. **How Belly Fat Reduction Leads to Better Energy Levels and Vitality**

Reducing belly fat is often associated with improved physical health, but its effects on energy levels and overall vitality are just as significant. Belly fat, particularly visceral fat (fat around the organs), can negatively impact metabolic function, hormone balance, and energy production. Here's how reducing belly fat leads to better energy and vitality, supported by scientific evidence.

1. Improved Insulin Sensitivity and Blood Sugar Regulation

Why It Works:

Excess belly fat, particularly visceral fat, is closely linked to insulin resistance, a condition where the body's cells become less responsive to insulin, leading to higher blood sugar levels and fatigue.

Scientific Evidence:

A study published in *Diabetes Care* found that abdominal fat reduction improved insulin sensitivity, helping to stabilize blood sugar levels. Stable blood sugar means more consistent energy levels and less energy crash throughout the day.

Practical Impact:

Less fatigue after meals.

Improved sustained energy throughout the day without the need for caffeine or sugar spikes.

2. Enhanced Hormonal Balance

Why It Works:

Visceral fat influences several hormones, including leptin (which regulates hunger) and cortisol (the stress hormone). High belly fat levels often lead to an imbalance in these hormones, which can increase hunger, stress, and fatigue.

Scientific Evidence:

Research published in *The Journal of Clinical Endocrinology & Metabolism* found that reducing belly fat led to significant improvements in hormonal regulation, including lower levels of cortisol and higher levels of leptin, helping to stabilize appetite and reduce stress.

Practical Impact:

Improved mood and reduced feelings of stress or anxiety.

More balanced energy throughout the day, with fewer cravings.

3. Increased Cardiovascular Health and Oxygen Flow

Why It Works:

Excess belly fat increases the risk of cardiovascular diseases, which can affect heart efficiency and oxygen delivery to tissues. Losing belly fat improves heart function, making it easier for oxygen and nutrients to circulate, boosting energy and vitality.

Scientific Evidence:

A 2018 study in *The American Journal of Physiology* showed that fat loss, particularly around the abdomen, resulted in improved cardiovascular health and increased VO2 max (a measure of cardiovascular fitness), which directly correlates to better energy levels.

Practical Impact:

Improved endurance and reduced fatigue during physical activity.

Better recovery time after exercise or daily tasks.

4. Better Sleep Quality

Why It Works:

Visceral fat can lead to sleep disturbances, including sleep apnea, which disrupts rest and reduces energy levels during the day. Reducing belly fat can improve sleep quality, leading to better recovery and increased vitality.

Scientific Evidence:

A study published in *Sleep* found that weight loss, particularly in the abdominal area, was associated with better sleep quality and fewer sleep disturbances.

Practical Impact:

Wake up feeling more refreshed and energized.

Enhanced mood and performance throughout the day due to improved sleep quality.

5. Improved Mental Clarity and Focus

Why It Works:

Belly fat influences systemic inflammation and brain function. Excess visceral fat can increase inflammation, which has been linked to cognitive decline and fatigue. Reducing belly fat helps lower inflammation, leading to better mental clarity and focus.

Scientific Evidence:

A study in *Brain, Behaviour, and Immunity* demonstrated that fat loss, particularly around the abdominal area, reduced markers of inflammation and improved cognitive function.

Practical Impact:
Increased mental clarity, focus, and productivity.

Better decision-making and reduced brain fog.

Takeaway
Reducing belly fat has far-reaching benefits beyond aesthetics. It improves insulin sensitivity, balances hormones, enhances cardiovascular function, boosts sleep quality, and reduces inflammation—all of which contribute to higher energy levels and greater vitality. By focusing on sustainable fat loss, you can experience a significant increase in overall well-being and sustained energy throughout your daily life.

Chapter 12: Building Healthy Habits for Long-Term Success

1. **Creating a Sustainable Fitness Routine: A Scientifically Proven Approach**

   Building a sustainable fitness routine is essential for long-term health and well-being. While quick-fix workouts or extreme regimes may offer short-term results, a sustainable routine ensures consistent progress and prevents burnout. Research supports that the most effective fitness plans are realistic, enjoyable, and adaptable to your life. Here's how to create a routine that you can stick to for the long haul.

   ## 1. Set Realistic and Achievable Goals

   Why It Works:

   Setting clear, attainable goals gives you a sense of direction and motivation. Unrealistic expectations can lead to frustration and burnout, while achievable goals encourage consistency and progress.

   Scientific Evidence:

   A study in *Psychological Bulletin* shows that people with specific and realistic goals are more likely to stick with their fitness routines. Goal-setting enhances commitment, especially when goals are broken into smaller, manageable steps.

   How to Do It:

   Break larger goals into smaller milestones (e.g., "**walk 30 minutes daily**" or "increase strength by lifting 5 more pounds").

Celebrate achievements to reinforce motivation.

2. Focus on Enjoyment and Variety

Why It Works:

When exercise is enjoyable, you're more likely to stick with it. Varying your routine also keeps it fresh and prevents monotony.

Scientific Evidence:

A study in *The Journal of Sport & Exercise Psychology* found that people who enjoy their workouts are more consistent and report higher levels of satisfaction. Additionally, variety prevents adaptation, keeping your body challenged and engaged.

How to Do It:

Try different activities—cycling, swimming, hiking, weightlifting, yoga—to find what you enjoy.

Switch up your routine every few weeks to avoid boredom and keep progress on track.

3. Incorporate Strength, Cardio, and Flexibility Training

Why It Works:

A balanced routine that includes strength training, cardiovascular exercise, and flexibility promotes overall fitness. Combining these elements improves endurance, builds muscle, and enhances mobility.

Scientific Evidence:

A 2016 review in *Sports Medicine* highlights the benefits of a balanced fitness program for overall health and injury prevention. Strength training builds lean muscle, while cardio improves heart health, and flexibility exercises enhance movement and prevent stiffness.

How to Do It:

Aim for at least 150 minutes of moderate-intensity cardio per week (e.g., brisk walking, cycling).

Include two or more days of strength training per week (e.g., bodyweight exercises or lifting weights).

Incorporate stretching or yoga for flexibility and recovery.

4. Start Slow and Gradually Increase Intensity

Why It Works:

Jumping into a high-intensity routine can lead to injury or burnout. Gradual progression allows your body to adapt and improves your chances of long-term success.

Scientific Evidence:

Research published in *The American Journal of Sports Medicine* shows that gradual progression reduces the risk of injury and helps maintain motivation by preventing overtraining and exhaustion.

How to Do It:

Begin with moderate-intensity workouts, and increase the duration, intensity, or weight incrementally.

Listen to your body—avoid pushing through pain or excessive fatigue.

5. Prioritize Consistency Over Intensity

Why It Works:

Regularity is key to building lasting habits. A sustainable routine is more about consistency than intensity. Exercising 3–4 times per week is far more beneficial than overexerting yourself for one week and quitting the next.

Scientific Evidence:

A study in *Frontiers in Psychology* shows that consistency is one of the strongest predictors of long-term fitness success. People who maintain regular activity, even at moderate intensity, experience better overall health than those who engage in sporadic, high-intensity exercise.

How to Do It:

Commit to a set schedule (e.g., work out every Monday, Wednesday, and Friday).

Focus on making exercise a non-negotiable part of your routine rather than something you "fit in" when convenient.

6. Prioritize Recovery and Rest

Why It Works:

Rest and recovery are essential components of a sustainable fitness routine. Without adequate recovery, overtraining can lead to fatigue, injury, and burnout.

Scientific Evidence:

A 2015 study in *Sports Medicine* shows that recovery, including sleep and rest days, is vital for muscle repair, hormone regulation, and preventing injury. Active recovery (e.g., walking, light stretching) is also important for maintaining flexibility and muscle function.

How to Do It:

Schedule rest days in between intense workouts.

Aim for 7–9 hours of quality sleep per night to support muscle recovery and energy levels.

Takeaway

A sustainable fitness routine is built on realistic goals, variety, consistency, and recovery. Focusing on what you enjoy and making gradual progress ensures that your routine becomes a lasting habit. By balancing different types of exercise, listening to your body, and taking time for recovery, you'll be able to maintain a routine that supports your long-term health and fitness goals.

2. **How to Integrate Healthy Eating into Your Lifestyle Long-Term**

Adopting healthy eating habits is key to maintaining long-term health, but it can be challenging to make these habits stick. The secret lies in making gradual changes, staying consistent, and finding a balance that fits your lifestyle. Here's how to integrate healthy eating into your daily routine, backed by scientific evidence.

1. Start Small and Make Gradual Changes

Why It Works:

Trying to overhaul your diet overnight is often unsustainable. Small, incremental changes are more likely to stick and can lead to lasting habits.

Scientific Evidence:

A 2012 study in *The American Journal of Clinical Nutrition* found that people who made gradual changes to their diets, such as reducing added sugars or incorporating more vegetables, were more successful at maintaining healthy eating patterns long-term.

How to Do It:

Start by replacing one unhealthy food with a healthier option each week. For example, swap sugary snacks for fruit or whole grains for refined carbs.

Focus on one area of your diet (like reducing processed foods or increasing fiber) rather than trying to change everything at once.

2. Plan Your Meals and Snacks

Why It Works:

Meal planning helps reduce decision fatigue, minimizes impulsive eating, and ensures you have healthy options readily available.

Scientific Evidence:

Research published in *The Journal of the Academy of Nutrition and Dietetics* suggests that meal planning is associated with better dietary intake, including higher consumption of fruits, vegetables, and whole grains.

How to Do It:

Plan your meals for the week, including snacks, and prep ingredients in advance.

Cook larger batches of healthy meals and store them for later to avoid unhealthy last-minute food choices.

3. Focus on Balanced, Nutrient-Dense Meals

Why It Works:

A balanced diet that includes a variety of nutrients supports overall health, energy levels, and satiety, reducing cravings and overeating.

Scientific Evidence:

A review in *Nutrients* showed that a diet rich in whole foods—fruits, vegetables, lean proteins, and healthy fats—improves long-term health outcomes, including reduced risk of chronic diseases like heart disease and diabetes.

How to Do It:

Include a source of lean protein (chicken, fish, legumes), healthy fats (avocado, nuts, olive oil), and fiber-rich carbs (whole grains, vegetables) in every meal.

Aim for a colorful plate, ensuring a variety of nutrients from different food groups.

4. Practice Mindful Eating

Why It Works:

Mindful eating encourages a greater awareness of hunger and fullness cues, preventing overeating and fostering a healthier relationship with food.

Scientific Evidence:

A study in *Appetite* found that practicing mindful eating led to reduced calorie intake, improved food choices, and better weight management.

How to Do It:

Eat without distractions (like phones or TV) and focus on the taste, texture, and enjoyment of your food.

Pause between bites to assess hunger levels, and stop eating when you feel satisfied, not full.

5. Allow Flexibility and Avoid Strict Restrictions

Why It Works:

Strict dieting can lead to feelings of deprivation, triggering overeating or binge eating. Flexibility helps prevent the "all-or-nothing" mindset and promotes long-term success.

Scientific Evidence:

Research in *The International Journal of Obesity* shows that flexible eating patterns, rather than rigid dieting, are linked to better long-term adherence and more sustainable weight management.

How to Do It:

Allow yourself occasional indulgences, but keep portions in check.

Balance treats with healthier choices throughout the week.

6. Stay Hydrated

Why It Works:

Proper hydration supports metabolism, digestion, and overall health, making it easier to make healthier food choices and feel energized.

Scientific Evidence:

A study published in *The Journal of Human Nutrition and Dietetics* found that adequate hydration can help control appetite and reduce the likelihood of mistaking thirst for hunger.

How to Do It:

Aim for at least 8 glasses (2 liters) of water a day, or more if you're physically active.

Start your day with water and hydrate before, during, and after meals to improve digestion and satiety.

7. Make Healthy Eating Social and Enjoyable

Why It Works:

Socializing around food can make healthy eating feel more rewarding and less isolating, improving adherence to dietary changes.

Scientific Evidence:

A 2019 study in *The Journal of Nutrition Education and Behaviour* found that people who engaged in social meal planning and cooking were more likely to stick to healthy eating habits.

How to Do It:

Cook meals with family or friends, making healthy eating a fun, communal activity.

Share your healthy recipes with others to create a support system and stay motivated.

Takeaway

Integrating healthy eating into your lifestyle long-term doesn't require drastic changes; it's about consistency, balance, and making small, sustainable adjustments. By focusing on nutrient-dense foods, planning ahead, staying hydrated, and practicing mindful eating, you can create a diet that not only supports your health goals but also fits seamlessly into you

Building Habits for a Balanced Life and Preventing Future Weight Gain

Preventing weight gain and maintaining a balanced lifestyle require long-term habits rather than short-term fixes. Research shows that small, consistent actions can create sustainable results, improving overall health and reducing the likelihood of regaining lost weight. Here's how to build habits that support balance and prevent future weight gain.

1. Prioritize Consistent Physical Activity

Why It Works:

Regular exercise not only burns calories but also boosts metabolism, improves mood, and helps maintain muscle mass, which is crucial for long-term weight management.

Scientific Evidence:

A 2014 study in *The American Journal of Preventive Medicine* found that individuals who engaged in regular physical activity were significantly less likely to experience weight regain after weight loss.

How to Do It:

1. Aim for at least 150 minutes of moderate-intensity exercise per week, such as brisk walking or cycling.

2. Incorporate strength training twice a week to build muscle, which increases resting metabolic rate.

2. Adopt a Balanced, Whole-Food Diet

Why It Works:

A diet rich in whole foods, such as fruits, vegetables, lean proteins, and healthy fats, provides essential nutrients and supports steady energy levels while reducing cravings for processed foods.

Scientific Evidence:

A 2020 review in *Advances in Nutrition* highlighted that diets focusing on whole, minimally processed foods are associated with better weight maintenance and lower risk of obesity.

How to Do It:

1. Use the 80/20 rule: eat nutrient-dense, whole foods 80% of the time, allowing 20% for indulgent treats.

2.   Focus on portion control, even with healthy foods, to avoid overeating.

3. Build a Healthy Relationship with Food

Why It Works:

Avoiding emotional eating and recognizing hunger cues can prevent overconsumption and help you develop a sustainable eating pattern.

Scientific Evidence:

Research in *Appetite* found that mindful eating practices, such as paying attention to hunger and satiety signals, reduce overeating and emotional eating behaviours.

How to Do It:

1.   Practice mindful eating by removing distractions during meals and savouring each bite.

2.   Learn to differentiate between physical hunger and emotional triggers like stress or boredom.

4. Get Quality Sleep

Why It Works:

Sleep deprivation disrupts hormones that regulate appetite, such as ghrelin (which increases hunger) and leptin (which signals fullness), leading to overeating.

Scientific Evidence:

A study in *Sleep Medicine Reviews* found that insufficient sleep is linked to increased caloric intake, reduced energy expenditure, and a higher risk of weight gain.

How to Do It:

1. Aim for 7–9 hours of quality sleep per night.

2. Establish a consistent sleep schedule by going to bed and waking up at the same time daily.

5. Manage Stress Effectively

Why It Works:

Chronic stress increases cortisol levels, which can lead to fat storage, particularly around the abdomen, and trigger cravings for high-calorie foods.

Scientific Evidence:

A 2018 study in *Psych neuroendocrinology* showed that stress management techniques, such as mindfulness and exercise, reduce cortisol levels and support healthier eating behaviours.

How to Do It:

1. Incorporate stress-reducing activities like meditation, yoga, or deep breathing into your daily routine.

2. Create boundaries for work and leisure to maintain a healthy work-life balance.

6. Monitor Progress Without Obsession

Why It Works:

Tracking your habits helps maintain awareness of your behaviours, but obsessing over numbers can create unnecessary stress.

Scientific Evidence:

A study in *Obesity* found that individuals who regularly monitored their weight and dietary habits were more likely to maintain their weight loss over time.

How to Do It:

1. Track your habits with a journal or app, focusing on consistency rather than perfection.

2. Measure progress using non-scale indicators like energy levels, mood, and how clothes fit.

7. Build a Support System

Why It Works:

Social connections foster accountability and encouragement, making it easier to stick to healthy habits.

Scientific Evidence:

A 2016 study in *Obesity Research & Clinical Practice* found that individuals with social support, such as friends or groups with similar goals, had better long-term weight management outcomes.

How to Do It:

1. Share your goals with friends or family who can encourage and motivate you.

2.   Consider joining fitness classes or support groups for a sense of community.

Takeaway

Building habits that support a balanced life and prevent future weight gain requires consistency, mindfulness, and a holistic approach. Focus on physical activity, balanced nutrition, quality sleep, and stress management to create a sustainable lifestyle. With patience and commitment, these habits will help you maintain your health and well-being for the long term.

Recap:

- Stop drinking chilled water or any chilled liquid from just now to put yourself on the tract of Fitness. Always prefer water or any drink on normal temperature or Luke warm.
- Drink Lemon Water on an empty stomach after you wake up in the morning.

How to Prepare Lemon Water

- Squeeze the juice of half a fresh lemon into a glass of lukewarm water.
- Drink it slowly on an empty stomach. Avoid adding sugar for maximum benefits.

Benefits of Drinking Lemon Water on an Empty Stomach

Lemon water has been celebrated for its health benefits when consumed first thing in the morning. Here's how it can support your overall well-being:

1. Boosts Digestion

- Stimulates the production of digestive enzymes, aiding in the breakdown of food.
- Helps relieve bloating, indigestion, and heartburn.

2. Detoxifies the Body

- Lemon water acts as a gentle cleanser, helping the liver flush out toxins.
- Encourages regular bowel movements and maintains a healthy digestive system.

3. Aids in Weight Loss

- Contains compounds like polyphenols that may suppress appetite and reduce fat accumulation.
- Drinking it can increase hydration, which supports metabolism and calorie burning.

4. Enhances Immunity

- Packed with vitamin C, which strengthens the immune system. Helps the body fight colds, flu, and other infections more effectively.

5. Improves Skin Health

- Vitamin C and antioxidants combat free radicals, reducing signs of aging like wrinkles.
- Promotes hydration, leading to clearer and healthier-looking skin.

6. Alkalizes the Body

- Despite its acidic taste, lemon creates an alkalizing effect in the body, balancing pH levels.
- A balanced pH may reduce inflammation and support overall health.

7. Freshens Breath

- Neutralizes Odor-causing bacteria in the mouth.
- Stimulates saliva production, which prevents dryness and bad breath.

8. Hydrates the Body

- Replenishes fluids after overnight dehydration.
- Adds flavour to water, encouraging increased water intake.

9. Supports Heart Health

- Rich in potassium, which supports healthy blood pressure levels.
- May improve circulation and cardiovascular health.

Note: While lemon water is beneficial, excessive consumption may erode tooth enamel or irritate the stomach for some individuals. Use a straw and rinse your mouth with plain water afterward to minimize dental risks.

- Walk everyday minimum 40-60 minutes: Jogging for 5 minutes followed by walking @5 KM/hour an average speed.
- Best time to go for walk is morning/evening/post dinner.
- Do some workout for 20-30 minutes:
- Some Strength workouts as mentioned in the book or you can consult your Gym trainer as well.
- Some Cardio workouts as mentioned in the book or you can consult your Gym trainer as well.
- Follow diet plan as mentioned in the Book.
- Do meditate after the workout followed by relaxation for few minutes. Link of some guided meditation are given in the additional resources page.

- Practice Breathing Techniques lie alternate nostril breathing. It's immensely beneficial to Body, Mind and Soul, Regular practice of breathing techniques helps in stabilizing your emotions & getting rid of negative thoughts as well.
- Do follow a minimum 20 minutes workout plan, you can follow a 20 minute workout plan suggested by the author on his personal channel https://www.youtube.com/watch?v=QGY9Cke8eqk

Motivation Tips:

- Develop a positive mindset about everything in your life which the foremost technique to overcome your health issues.
- If you are surrounded with people with negative mindset or negative habits try to replace them with people with positive mindset and positive habits.
- Think like if you have accumulated extra fat in your belly due to some bad life style habits, then the same can be cured as well by improving/changing those habits in life. Wish You all the best

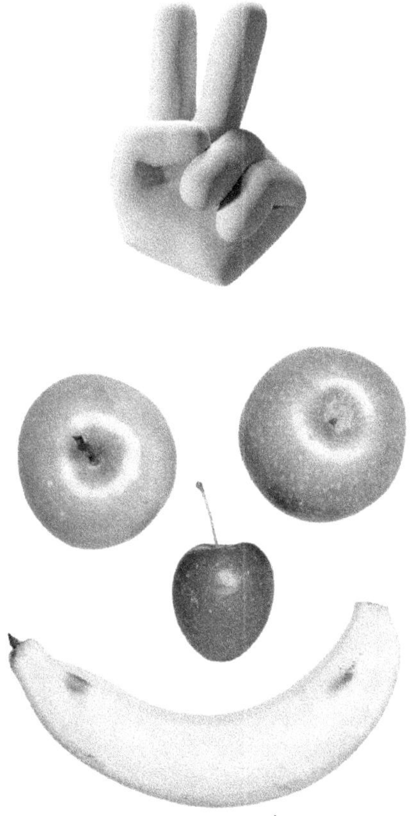

30 Day Fitness Tracker

Day 1

Flatten Your Belly, Transform Your Life

30 Day Fitness Tracker

Day 2

Flatten Your Belly, Transform Your Life

30 Day Fitness Tracker

Day 3

Flatten Your Belly, Transform Your Life

30 Day Fitness Tracker

Day 4

Flatten Your Belly, Transform Your Life

30 Day Fitness Tracker

Day 5

Flatten Your Belly, Transform Your Life

30 Day Fitness Tracker

Day 6

Flatten Your Belly, Transform Your Life

30 Day Fitness Tracker

Day 7

Flatten Your Belly, Transform Your Life

30 Day Fitness Tracker

Day 8

Flatten Your Belly, Transform Your Life

30 Day Fitness Tracker

Day 9

Flatten Your Belly, Transform Your Life

30 Day Fitness Tracker

Day 10

Flatten Your Belly, Transform Your Life

30 Day Fitness Tracker

Day 11

Flatten Your Belly, Transform Your Life

30 Day Fitness Tracker

Day 12

Flatten Your Belly, Transform Your Life

30 Day Fitness Tracker

Day 13

Flatten Your Belly, Transform Your Life

30 Day Fitness Tracker

Day 14

Flatten Your Belly, Transform Your Life

30 Day Fitness Tracker

Day 15

Flatten Your Belly, Transform Your Life

30 Day Fitness Tracker

Day 16

Flatten Your Belly, Transform Your Life

30 Day Fitness Tracker

Day 17

Flatten Your Belly, Transform Your Life

30 Day Fitness Tracker

Day 18

Flatten Your Belly, Transform Your Life

30 Day Fitness Tracker

Day 19

Flatten Your Belly, Transform Your Life

30 Day Fitness Tracker

Day 20

Flatten Your Belly, Transform Your Life

30 Day Fitness Tracker

Day 21

Flatten Your Belly, Transform Your Life

30 Day Fitness Tracker

Day 22

Flatten Your Belly, Transform Your Life

30 Day Fitness Tracker

Day 23

Flatten Your Belly, Transform Your Life

30 Day Fitness Tracker

Day 24

Flatten Your Belly, Transform Your Life

30 Day Fitness Tracker

Day 25

Flatten Your Belly, Transform Your Life

30 Day Fitness Tracker

Day 26

Flatten Your Belly, Transform Your Life

30 Day Fitness Tracker

Day 27

Flatten Your Belly, Transform Your Life

30 Day Fitness Tracker

Day 28

Flatten Your Belly, Transform Your Life

30 Day Fitness Tracker

Day 29

Flatten Your Belly, Transform Your Life

30 Day Fitness Tracker

Day 30